Date Due			
OCT 15 1991			
OCT 1 5 1991			
MAR 08 1995			
MAR 1 5 1995			
JAN 0 2 1996			
JAN 0 9 1996			

DANCE
CANADA

DANCE CANADA

AN ILLUSTRATED HISTORY

MAX WYMAN

Douglas & McIntyre
Vancouver/Toronto

Douglas & McIntyre Ltd.
1615 Venables Street
Vancouver, British Columbia   V5L 2H1

Canadian Cataloguing in Publication Data
Wyman, Max, 1939–
    Dance Canada
    Includes index.
    ISBN 0-88894-657-0
    1. Dancing – Canada – History.   I. Title.
GV162.W95 1989   793.3'2'0971   C89-091364-1

Editor: Saeko Usukawa
Design by Barbara Hodgson and Alexandra Hass
Front jacket photograph by David Street
Back jacket photograph by Edouard Lock
Typeset by The Typeworks
Printed and bound in Canada by Hemlock Printers Ltd.

All care has been taken to trace ownership of images in this book. Omissions will be corrected in subsequent editions, provided notification is sent to the publisher.

—— For my father,
Frederick Wyman,
who taught the significance of what went before

Contents

Preface

The past is a foreign country; they do things differently there.
L. P. Hartley, *The Go-Between*

In a period rich in dance and dancing, it is difficult to understand properly the bravery with which the pioneers of dancing in Canada tackled the challenges that confronted them, or to appreciate fully the extent of their achievements.

This should not dim their glories. Time may have blurred the detail, but the canvas on which the picture of Canadian dance is painted is broad. Tackling the telling of this story is like exploring that canvas with the lights out and only a candle flame to show the way.

This book is neither an academic treatise nor a person-by-person, moment-by-moment record of everything that has taken place in Canadian dance. What it attempts is an illumination of the most significant outlines of context, influence, action and effect in the development of theatrical dancing in Canada.

Folk dance, social dance, the dance of Canada's native peoples, dance teaching and dance on film and television (all important topics in themselves) are touched on only briefly; and the section dealing with the seventeenth to nineteenth centuries is a beginning only.

The story told here is told without varnish—it would be doing the groundbreakers less than dignity to smooth away the wrinkles and flush the cheeks like some paid portraitist—but it is also told with affection and regard. The story of dancing in Canada is a story of the interplay of individual personalities of many types and temperaments; it can also be seen as a metaphor for the development of Canada itself—the gradual evolution, against all odds and in the face of two colonizing cultures, of a body of activity unique to this northern place.

I write, of course, from a personal viewpoint; but what I have written would not have been possible without the help of many individuals. It was Iris Garland, at Simon Fraser University, who planted the seed, when I spoke about Canadian dance history to her students in the late 1970s. The timeliness of her idea can be measured by the enthusiasm this project has generated throughout the lengthy period of research, and by the extent of assistance and information that has in almost every case been readily and generously provided by the individuals involved.

The founders of the country's three senior ballet companies—Gweneth Lloyd and Betty Farrally, Celia Franca and Ludmilla Chiriaeff—gave lavishly of their time and were frank and patient in response to my extensive questioning.

I was also fortunate to obtain valuable perspectives from many dancers, choreographers, administrators, writers and academics—among them David Adams, Lawrence Adams, Miriam Adams, Carol Anderson, Reid Anderson, Joanne Ashe, Janet Baldwin, Patricia Beatty, Sally Brayley Bliss, Peter Boneham, Michel Boudot, Rachel Browne, Erik Bruhn, Duncan Cameron, Norman Campbell, Ruth Carse, Barbara Clausen, Susan Cohen, Cliff Collier, Michael Crabb, George Crum, Christopher Dafoe, Nancy Lima Dent, Rosemary Deveson, Sir Anton

Dolin, Margaret Dragu, David Earle, Ernst Eder, Lee Eisler, Martine Epoque, Michèle Febvre, Dick Foose, Maria Formolo, Paul-André Fortier, Patricia Fraser, Denise Fujiwara, Anne-Marie Gaston, Arthur Gelber, Eva von Gencsy, Margie Gillis, Lawrence Gradus, Alexander Grant, Nelson Gray, Fernau Hall, Gertrud and Magda Hanova, Dorothy Harris, Evelyn Hart, Vanessa Harwood, Eric Hehner, Karen Jamieson, Roger Jones, Henny Jurriens, Karen Kain, John Kelly, Daniel Léveillé, Cathy Levy, Marianne Livant, Edouard Lock, Uriel Luft, David Y. H. Lui, Alexander MacDougall, Colin McIntyre, Susan McKenzie, Susan Macpherson, Andrée Millaire, Judith Marcuse, Richard Marcuse, Dianne Miller, David Moroni, John Neumeier, Duncan Noble, Selma Landen Odom, Jacqueline Ogg, Betty Oliphant, Jean Stoneham Orr, Brydon Paige, Kenny Pearl, David Peregrine, Jean-Pierre Perreault, Hugh Pickett, Linda Rabin, Renald Rabu, Peter Randazzo, Paula Ravitz, Jeanne Renaud, Françoise Riopelle, Allan Risdill, Tedd Robinson, Paula Ross, Geneviève Salbaing, Elsie Salomons, Sekai, Lynn Seymour, Wynne Shaw, Lois Smith, Daniel Soulières, Arnold Spohr, Grant Strate, Françoise Sullivan, Charlene Tarver, Iro Tembeck, Veronica Tennant, Lauretta Thistle, Jean Harper Tilley, Nesta Toumine, Jack Udashkin, Keith Urban, Kee Van Deurs, Norbert Vesak, Kati Vita, Diana Vorps, Vincent Warren, Herbert Whittaker, Valerie Wilder, Sonja Barton Woods, Anna Wyman and David Yeddeau.

I owe a special debt of gratitude to certain other researchers involved in Canadian dance history. Michael Crabb's short historical text for *Dance Today in Canada* (published with Andrew Oxenham in 1976) made a useful point of departure. My section on June Roper and Vancouver in the late 1930s owes much to the patient researches of Leland Windreich, who generously allowed me to draw freely on materials gathered for his work in progress on the eight Vancouver dancers who went to the Ballets Russes. Karen Greenhough kindly allowed me to hear a number of taped interviews she conducted with Vancouver dance pioneers. Barbara Scales, in Montreal, provided consultation on the career of Seda Zaré, drawn from her work in progress on that dancer's life. The tireless Pierre Guilmette, at the library of the Université Laval, was a great source of encouragement and assistance, particularly in the area of the seventeenth and nineteenth centuries. Jillian Officer and her staff (Robyn Gallimore in particular) at the Dictionary of Dance project at the University of Waterloo helped to check and amplify data.

I was fortunate to be able to call on the records and experience of Sydney Johnson, who wrote about dance for the Montreal *Star*, for valuable information about the growth of dance in Montreal. Robert B. Todd's articles in *Vandance* provided information on visitors to Vancouver in the early twentieth century. Research assistance was also provided by Heather McCallum and her staff at the theatre department at the Toronto Metropolitan Library; Hugh A. Dempsey and his staff at the Glenbow Museum in Calgary; Nancy J. Hurn at the Canadian National Exhibition archives; Patricia Ekland, co-ordinator of *Creative Canada* at the University of Victoria; Mark Porteous and Mike Bigold at the Royal Winnipeg Ballet; and Jennifer Mascall.

I am grateful, too, for the assistance provided by the publicists at Canada's dance companies—prominent among them Lendre Rodgers Stearns and Mary

Bashaw at the Royal Winnipeg Ballet; Marcia McClung, Roz Gray, Greg Patterson and Willo Solomon at the National Ballet of Canada; and Irene Malyholowka at Les Grands Ballets Canadiens.

Help on points of detail came from Janet Judd at the Royal Ballet in London; Doreen Scouler of the Royal Academy of Dancing in Canada; Vanessa Lindsay, editor of *Dance Gazette* in London; Sarah C. Woodcock at the Victoria and Albert Museum, London; John Merritt at CBC Radio, Vancouver; Claude Gosselin at the Musée d'art contemporain in Montreal; Judy Malone at the Art Gallery of Ontario; B. C. Cuthbertson, public records archivist for Nova Scotia; Jean l'Espérance at the National Archives of Canada; and Suzanne Blier Cantin.

The Canada Council provided a grant that enabled me to take a year away from my duties as columnist and critic at the Vancouver *Province* and to travel to undertake the necessary research, and I express my gratitude for that valuable help. However, while the Council's dance staff past and present—notably Monique Michaud, Barbara Laskin, Holly Gnaedinger and Richard Rutherford—were unstinting in their assistance and co-operation, and while I inevitably deal with the Council's role in the development of dance in Canada, I neither wish nor pretend to be a spokesman for the Council, or a representative of its views.

My thanks go, too, to Dona Harvey, former managing editor at *The Province*, and her successor, Bob McMurray, for their ongoing support for the project overall.

I am particularly grateful to my editor at Douglas & McIntyre, Saeko Usukawa, for her intelligent and sympathetic approach to the task of textual abridgement.

None of it would have been possible, however, without the constant support and assistance of Susan Mertens, whose candid assessments have given the book amplitude, and whose unflagging belief in the project's ultimate worth helped keep it alive in dark days.

M. W., Lions Bay, June 1989

DANCE
CANADA

Introduction

Touring northern Canada with the now-defunct Regina Modern Dance Works sometime in the 1970s, Maria Formolo, a dancer and choreographer, fell into conversation with the janitor at a school where the company had been playing.

"I don't want to hurt your feelings," he said, "but I don't think you people are very good dancers. You practise every day, but it's still not as good as what dancers did in the old days. Can you make the rain come?"

———

The Canadian scholar and critic Northrop Frye, writing about what he terms a feeling "more Canadian than English" in certain Old English poems, has referred to the "terrible isolation of the creative mind" in a thinly settled country under a bleak northern sky.

The pioneers of theatre dancing in Canada knew that terrible isolation well. They numbered not much more than a handful to begin with, and they were scattered across the face of the second-largest country on earth. Few of them were native-born Canadians. Until as late as the 1970s, leadership in dance in Canada was almost exclusively in the hands of immigrants, initially from Europe, later from the United States. Most of them were women.

The companies themselves were often small gatherings of enthusiasts grouped around a visionary individual. And when we talk of companies existing in Canada at that time, we are talking not of some kind of early National Ballet or Toronto Dance Theatre, but of small, often quite disorganized groups of amateur enthusiasts. There is no record of paid performance until the 1940s, and even then the payment was a pittance—$3 a show at the early Winnipeg Ballet. People danced because they loved it, or because they believed in the work, and they invested their time and their energies without thought of recompense. Until well into the second half of this century, the first thing Canadian dancers did if they had their sights set on an international career was leave the country, usually under an assumed name.

The disconnectedness was acute. The Canadian Ballet Festival movement in the early 1950s began to open up communication, but it was not until the inception of the Dance in Canada Association in the early 1970s that dancers and choreographers in Canada began to form any clear idea of what was happening in their art form in parts of the country other than their own.

In the mid-1950s, a great debate was raging about the cultural future of Canada. Vincent Massey's Royal Commission on National Development in the Arts, Letters and Sciences had reported its views on "what can make our country great, and what can make it one," CBC television and the Stratford Festival were new in the land, and the creation of the Canada Council was imminent.

In the winter 1954 edition of *Queen's Quarterly*, Guy Glover, a National Film Board producer and ballet enthusiast, wrote: "Canadian ballet stands today at a kind of crossroads. Will Canadian dance artists move off down the road well-trodden by the big international companies . . . the road of a ready-made idiom, of largely ready-made ideas and of a ready-made taste? Or will Canadian ballet branch off into the seemingly dangerous (because unmapped) territory of technical discovery and new subject-matter—in an attempt to fashion an idiom and a taste of its own?"

What Canadian dance did was go in both directions at once. In a nation where pluralism was to become official policy, perhaps it could hardly do otherwise. Whether it has succeeded in fashioning "an idiom and a taste of its own" remains a matter for conjecture.

——

Dances have been made on Canadian themes for almost five decades, without noticeably changing the way Canadians think and feel about themselves. The record goes back at least as far as Boris Volkoff's Eskimo legend *Mala* and his Indian-inspired *Mon-ka-ta* in 1936, and Gweneth Lloyd's little fables on Prairie life, *Grain* and *Kilowatt Magic*, three years later. Often, it was simply a matter of translating folk tales into narrative dance—Ruth Sorel's *La Gaspésienne*, Volkoff's *The Red Ear of Corn* (both in 1949), and a variety of versions of both Louis Hémon's novel *Maria Chapdelaine* and the legend of *Rose Latulippe*, the Quebec girl who danced with the devil. There have been many *divertissements* using Canadian (generally French-Canadian) music and locales (Brian Macdonald's *Tam Ti Delam* in 1974 and *Hangman's Reel* in 1978, for instance). Less often, attempts have been made to penetrate the folksy surface and make a theatrical statement about particularly Canadian concerns: Gweneth Lloyd's *Shadow on the Prairie* (1952), dealing with the fatal homesickness of an immigrant woman; Anna Wyman's *Klee Wyck: A Ballet for Emily* (1975), about the artist Emily Carr's closeness to the people and landscapes of the West Coast; Ann Ditchburn's *Nelligan* (1975), evoking the spirit of the Québécois poet; Maria Formolo's *Winter-piece Suite* (1979), reacting to the work of the Prairie artist William Kurelek; Macdonald's *Etapes* (1982), dealing with Quebec independence and the loosening of standards in Canadian society; Karen Jamieson's *Rainforest* (1987), exploring the force of myth and magic in West Coast Indian society.

There was even, for a time, an entire company devoted to Canadian themes and the performance of traditional dance, Les Feux-Follets. Founded in the early 1950s by a Montreal anthropologist, Michel Cartier, the company turned professional in 1964, and its collection of Canadian dance materials—among them a dance donated by the Kwakiutl Indian chief Mungo Martin—became the focus for a theatrical spectacular along the lines of the hugely popular touring European folk ensembles of the 1960s and 1970s. However, it collapsed a decade later, having degenerated under a new director into tourist bureau glitter and nightclub ethnic populism.

——

Within the choreographic community of Canada, we have a core of creators who have developed individual identities in their dance-making. There is nothing recognizably Canadian about their work. Personal expressiveness is a far cry from nationalist representation. But the obsession to identify ourselves as a nation remains; acutely aware of the giant at our shoulder, we are sometimes tempted to believe that the mere proclamation of our name will tell us who we are. Canadian dance is a bringing-together of many different and often seemingly mismatched elements—the choreographic version of that most popular of all images for the Canadian identity, the mosaic.

Canada has always had an openness to other influences, a willingness to bear another's imprint. Much is able to flourish in Canada's atmosphere of amiable hospitality and uncompetitive co-operation that might find survival hard elsewhere. Dance that is made in Canada characteristically lacks New York's frantic, nervy urbanity. A sense of innocence and of unwillingness to assert permeate this story, and if we seek an identity in Canadian dance, we might most usefully look for it here—in the unassuming dedication to the art of dancing that wafts like a perfumed cloud off the stage and into the hearts of audiences wherever the Royal Winnipeg Ballet performs; in the heart-on-sleeve romanticism, almost touching in its naiveté, of some of the Montreal modernists; in the brute determination that allowed Gweneth Lloyd and Betty Farrally and Celia Franca and Ludmilla Chiriaeff to do the things they did because they did not know they could not be done; in the enduring innocence and sense of wonder that shines from the individual who guided the Royal Winnipeg Ballet to international triumphs, Arnold Spohr—the first native-born Canadian to be trusted with the leadership of a significant Canadian arts institution.

The influences that dominated the development of Canadian dance are the influences that dominated the growth of the country: two colonizing cultures, the inhibiting force in Quebec of a conservative church, massive immigration (with all its baggage) from Europe, and cultural overspill from the United States.

Those who settled the cultural soil came much later than those who settled the physical wilderness, but they shared with their predecessors the entirely human tendency to make, in their new home, not new models but echoes of what they had known before. The Canadians who launched the National Ballet of Canada made no secret of the fact that what they wanted was another Sadler's Wells company, for Canada, and they went to the Sadler's Wells founder, Ninette de Valois, for advice on how to get it. Much later the American influence was to come striding across the border, all push and hope and iconoclasm. And what has evolved in dance in Canada is a unique, often very appealing twining of those two main cultural threads that bind Canada—European formality and seriousness, and America's nonconformist vitality.

Outside Quebec it has been rare to come across Canadian artists who speak in a passionate way about issues that pertain uniquely to the country or to the people who inhabit it—and on the occasions when it happened in Quebec (the publication of *refus global* in 1948 and the emergence of the Quebec dance experimentalists two decades later), the thrust evolved from essentially similar circumstances: a desire on the part of artists to make statements that would comment on and establish their separateness from the society in which they were working.

What the evidence of Quebec makes clear is that while the development of dance in Canada is locked into history, it is also locked into location. When we want to know who we are, as Frye points out, it is useful first to know *where* we are, and the debate over regionalism versus federalism remains a hot one.

This debate has from time to time given rise to concern among those who have assumed responsibility for its support. In the early 1980s, the federal government flirted with the view that true excellence in the arts could only be fostered by bringing together in certain central places enough artistic activity to generate a climate in which excellence could thrive. On a similar argument, a decade earlier, unsuccessful demands were made for the nomination of the National Ballet School in Toronto as the official centre of excellence and guardian of standards for the teaching of ballet throughout Canada; even earlier than that, for reasons that also included the economic, there were proposals to coalesce the three major ballets into one truly *national* company. But as the world began to come to terms with living in McLuhan's village, as ideas became the *esperanto* of art, common property and effortlessly assimilable, the pre-eminence of the major centres diminished, and the unique cultural power of the region, the town, the neighbourhood, the domestic circle—its rootedness in the specifics of human life out of which the universals spring—began to reassert itself. Dancers no longer needed to leave the country to become famous; they did not even need to leave home.

Today, Canadians have available elements of virtually every human dance form. In the area of nonprofessional performance, folk dance is plentiful, much of it surviving in the clubs and societies of immigrant nationalities, and a number of groups, notably the Shumka Ukrainian Dancers, in Edmonton, have attempted to establish professional touring ensembles.

The dance of Canada's native peoples is more difficult to find in its authentic form, though a recent reawakening of interest in native Indian arts has led to its improved preservation, at a high level of accuracy. Many dances are still "possessed" by individuals and passed down a family for generations, and often they are still in use for their original ceremonial purposes. And while there has been little attempt to integrate Indian dance-forms with Western theatrical dancing, there have been attempts to mount authentic Indian dance in a theatrical format: the K'san dancers from Hazelton in northern British Columbia, for instance, travel outside their immediate environment to show their dance and music heritage to a wider, predominantly white audience.

We are only slowly seeing the emergence of a true independence of creative thought in Canadian choreography—an art that, in its combination of subject and style, is national without being nationalist. But Canada is slowly beginning to produce dancers and choreographers whose work not only speaks for itself but ranks, by international agreement, with the world's most exciting, not only in ballet but across the full range of modern and experimental dance. The terrible isolation of the creative mind has become part of Canada's history.

The future remains unpredictable. The flood of new Canadians from Europe has slowed; Canada's artists are finally coming to terms with the cultural overspill from the south; but the flood of new Canadians from Africa, India, the Caribbean, Asia and the Orient continues to swell. And it is surely in its continuing openness to that diversity, that plurality, that ambiguity, and in the tolerance and mutual regard that such diversity exacts, that Canadian dance is most likely to discover its identity.

BEGINNINGS : *1534–1900*

Beginnings

Jacques Cartier's journal of 1534 records an encounter in the Baie des Châleurs with seven canoes bearing "wild men," all dancing "and making many signs of joy and mirth, as it were desiring our friendship." By the shore, women sang and danced in the water. Cartier's journals provide the first written record of dancing in Canada, but it was not until Marc Lescarbot published his *History of New France* in 1609 that any kind of detailed records were made of the kind of dancing that was performed.

The Indians of New France dance for four reasons, wrote Lescarbot—to please their gods, to cheer someone up, to rejoice in victory or to prevent sickness. "Lascivious pleasure," he noted, "has not yet so far prevailed upon them as to make them dance at its bidding, a thing which should serve as a lesson to Christians."

Lescarbot was a Parisian lawyer, and a member of a party that explorer Samuel de Champlain led from the French colony at Port Royal (now Annapolis Royal, Nova Scotia). The dances were all performed, said Lescarbot, in the round, "and they dance vehemently, striking the ground with their feet, and springing up in a half-leap . . . to be more nimble, they commonly strip stark naked, because their dresses of skins hinder them; and if they have any heads or arms of their enemies, they carry them about their necks, dancing with this fair jewel which they will sometimes bite, so great is their hatred even against the dead."

To Lescarbot, these rituals must have seemed exotic and strange. But he was a thoughtful man, with a wide range of classical reference, and he saw a number of parallels between what he saw the Indians do and the fashions in dancing that were current at home. The *ballet de cour*, which had evolved from the court masquerades and pastorals of the Italian Renaissance, was still a social diversion in Paris. In 1581 the court in Paris saw what was effectively the first ballet, the *Ballet comique de la reine*, created by Balthasar de Beaujoyeux. Its significance lay in what it suggested was possible in terms of the integration of many elements—action, music, scenery, machinery, costume, dance and verse.

Lescarbot himself presented a masque, *The Theatre of Neptune*, on the waters of the harbour at Port Royal in 1606. Staged to celebrate the return of the colony's leader from an expedition down the Acadian coast, it may have been the first European attempt at large-scale dramatic or balletic public performance in the Americas, outside the Spanish colonies, far to the south.

————

Throughout the early seventeenth century, dance in France stagnated. With the reign of Louis XIV came the beginnings of an understanding of dance's value as an art form. Dance was no longer a mere *divertissement* between the scenes of a play or an opera, but was to become an integral part of the work itself.

In the colonies of new France, thousands of miles across the Atlantic, the force of these developments was slow to be felt.

The Jesuit Relations, a regular series of reports from missionaries to the Mother Church in France, record a number of theatrical presentations in the middle seventeenth century—a tragicomedy in 1640 in Quebec City, to honour the birth of the new dauphin; a production of Corneille's *Le Cid* in 1646; and, also in 1646, "a kind of ballet—to wit, five soldiers," performed at the marriage of Montpellier, a soldier and a shoemaker, to the daughter of Sevestre. In February of 1647 a ballet was given at the warehouse of the Company of One Hundred Associates, but the Jesuits reported that "not one of our fathers or brethren was present." The Catholic church, Quebec society's backbone, disapproved of all forms of dancing—an influence that extended well into the twentieth century.

When the British assumed power following the Treaty of Paris in 1763, official restraints against dancing and public entertainment were loosened, but this was not much more than an official recognition of prevailing conditions. Theatrical performance had become frequent; by the late eighteenth century, Montreal had seven spaces for public performance.

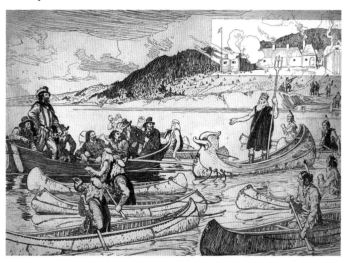

The *Quebec Gazette* of October 24, 1765, announced performances by a troupe called Les Villageoises Canadiennes—a comedy, a ballet of shepherds and shepherdesses, and character dances by three dancers "who have always been applauded in this part of North America." Admission cost 20 shillings, but 20 free tickets were set aside for "maiden ladies who do not have resources enough to amuse themselves but would like to do so." The *Gazette* also mentions a comic pastoral dance to be given in December 1783.

Generally regarded as the first play staged in Canada, Marc Lescarbot's masque, The Theatre of Neptune, *took place on the waters of the harbour of Port Royal in 1606. Looking on from the shore and from canoes as Neptune greeted the colony's returning leader were the people of local Chief Membertou. (C. W. Jefferys drawing, National Archives of Canada, C-106968)*

By this time, the professional ballerina had emerged in Europe. Marie Sallé had significantly expanded the potential for dramatic expressiveness in dance (and scandalized the citizenry) when she abandoned the traditional face mask and danced in day clothes in 1719. But when Sallé's great rival, Marie-Anne de Cupis de Camargo, shortened her skirts by an all-important few inches in the 1730s—a gesture that, in allowing her audiences to see the delicacy of her footwork, multiplied at a stroke the possibilities of technique in performance—she was regarded by some as a heretic.

John Durang, the first American to become famous as a professional dancer, arrived in Canada in 1797 with the Ricketts Circus of Philadelphia, the first circus to appear in Canada. Durang became fascinated by Indian life during his Canadian visit, and records in his autobiography, *The Memoir of John Durang, American Actor, 1785–1816*, that he "got up an Indian characteristic dance."

"I had my own dress which I purchased from an Indian for rum. The dances I learned from some Chipeway and Naudowessie chiefs of the West . . . I performed the Pipe Dance; the manner is gracefull and pleasing in the nature of savage harmony. Next, the Eagle Tail Dance. I concluded with the War Dance, descriptive of their exploits, throwing myself in different postures with firm steps with hatchet and knife, representing the manner they kill and scalp and take prisoners with the yells and war whoops."

By 1830 the emphasis on allegory and classicism that had dominated ballet had been replaced by an interest in recognizable themes and individuals: the rise of the Romantic movement in ballet had begun. In the colonies, meanwhile, both indigenous and imported dance attractions had been steadily gaining importance.

Alexandre Placide, renowned for the attractiveness of the girls in his *corps de ballet*, presented *The Bird Catcher* at Halifax in 1799 (Durang had presented it in Montreal the previous year); and in 1819 Placide's son Henry visited Halifax to dance in *The Miraculous Mill or The Old Ground Young*.

Montreal at this period saw works like *The Tars of Old England* and *The Scots Milliners* by a former London ballet master and dancer, Cipriani, who stayed on to open a dancing academy. And Dauberval's enormously popular ballet, *La Fille mal gardée*, given its premiere in France in 1789, was introduced to Canada in 1816, in Quebec City. (Over 150 years later, it became a handsome addition to the repertoire of the National Ballet of Canada.)

By the 1820s there is evidence of a Canadian dancer, perhaps the first, establishing a regular touring outlet across the border. This was Mme. S. Aspinall, an English dancer who set up in Quebec City in 1820 as a teacher, claiming to have been taught by Auguste Vestris, son of Gaetano, each known in his turn by the Paris public as "le dieu de la danse." Aspinall gave solo performances at Quebec City in 1824 and 1825, before embarking on annual presentations in New York.

There is no record of visits to Canada by the great European dancers of the Romantic era—Marie Taglioni, Fanny Elssler, Carlotta Grisi—nor by the early American women stars, Augusta Maywood and Mary Ann Lee. But Céleste Keppler, better known as Mme. Céleste, a French dancer, visited Quebec City in 1829, and played there and in Montreal during her triumphant tour of North America in 1835. It was during that tour that she gave American audiences their first sight of *La Sylphide*, the 1832 ballet that launched Romanticism in dance; *The French Spy*, a spectacular about the conquest of Algiers; and an extract from Auber's *Le Dieu et la bayadère* (*The Maid of Cashmere*), created in 1830 for the originator of *La Sylphide*, Taglioni.

A highlight of Canadian entertainment in 1847 and 1848 was the visit of a group of 48 children from Vienna, Les Petites Danseuses Viennoises. Houses were packed with admirers. "If dancing, as someone has said, is the poetry of motion," wrote a reviewer in the *Montreal Transcript*, "this is the poetry of poetry."

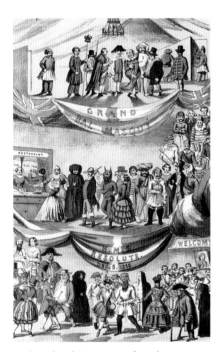

A Grand Bal Masque on board H.M.S. Resolute, *5 December 1850, by G. F. McDougall for the* Illustrated London News, *11 December 1850. (National Archives of Canada, C-28266)*

The adoration of the Romantically poetic in ballet rapidly declined as the world gathered speed in the second half of the nineteenth century. By the 1860s balletic performance in Europe had degenerated to the level of tricks, novelty and theatrical spectaculars. Ballet's main focus shifted to Russia. Dancing had been taught at the Imperial School of Ballet in St. Petersburg since 1734, and a succession of French and French-taught ballet-masters had developed the Russian repertoire and style. Europe was considered so superior in dance at this time that Russians would Europeanize their names—just as, in the 1930s, Canadian and U.S. dancers seeking extra cachet would Russianize theirs.

The most influential of these imports was Marius Petipa, a Frenchman who forged the basic form of classical ballet as we know it today. Petipa assigned prime importance to the choreography, relegating music to a supporting role (though there is nothing secondary about much of the music Tchaikovsky wrote for him), and he built his ballets according to certain "classic" principles of structure and composition. It is from this period that some of ballet's most enduring masterpieces (*Swan Lake, The Nutcracker, The Sleeping Beauty*) derive.

In North America, the move away from Romanticism is generally dated from the 1866 production of *The Black Crook*, an elaborate spectacle-extravaganza that sowed the seeds of a form that was rapidly to degenerate into an equally popular entertainment of its own—vaudeville.

Spectacle and easy diversion became paramount; style and subtlety yielded priority to theatricality and exotica. The American performer Loie Fuller did her *Fire Dance* at the Vancouver Opera House in 1896, and dazzled a capacity audience with her manipulated lights and her swirling silks, if not with her footwork.

It was on the vaudeville circuit that Ruth St. Denis and Ted Shawn showed their commercialized Eastern exotica to Canada on frequent visits between 1914 and 1924. (Dancing alongside St. Denis and Doris Humphrey in the *Siamese Ballet* in 1917 was an early Canadian ballet export, Edna Malone, who had left her home in Nelson, B.C., to study at the Denishawn school in Los Angeles.)

Spectaculars were a favourite form of entertainment in Toronto. The Misses Sternberg, who taught dancing (including classical training) and physical culture to Toronto society girls, staged large-scale spectaculars as early as 1900. The grandstand pageant at the Canadian National Exhibition every summer was always a guaranteed draw, with fireworks and a thrilling burning, and acres of dancing bodies.

Anna Pavlova made the first of four Vancouver appearances during her first North American tour in 1910, in partnership with Mikhail Mordkin, and the thing that drew greatest approval from the local critic was the "world of unreality" created by the pair of them in her *Bacchanale*.

The American writer Marcia Siegel argues that Pavlova was significant to the beginnings of modern dance in the U.S. through her example to women that it was possible for an artist to survive and thrive outside the male-dominated ballet-company hierarchies.

But her significance in Canada (which she visited often) was chiefly as an inspiration to dance. It does not matter that, in today's terms, her material was conservative kitsch and her choreography was, from all accounts and records, narrow and self-serving. The freshness and spontaneity of her dancing inspired the young performers in Canada's audiences with a dream of artistic perfection. Jean Tilley, a Sternberg pupil, recalled that, with the advent of Pavlova, "for the first time the boring barre exercises made sense. We induced graceful rhythm into our stilted bodies."

But Anna Pavlova was an exception. In the early part of the twentieth century, art dance, in Canada as everywhere, was in a slump.

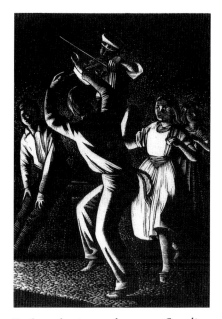

By the early nineteenth century, Canadians were dancing a lively mix of square dances, jigs, reels and clogs, often to the accompaniment of the fiddle. One of the most popular of these dances was the Red River Jig, depicted in a woodcut by Walter Joseph Phillips (1884–1963). (Copyright the estate of W. J. Phillips, National Archives of Canada, C-110879)

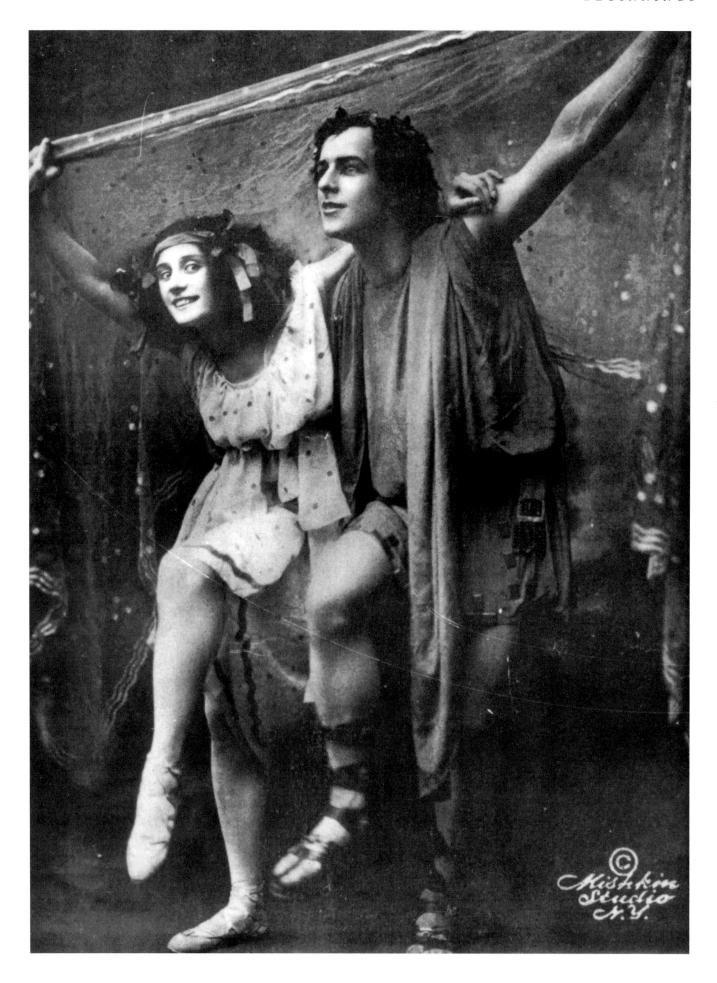

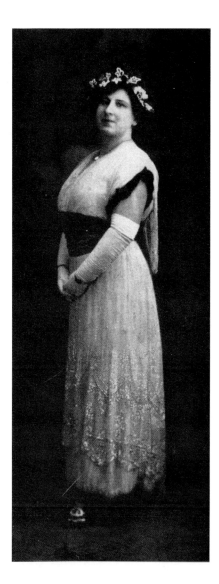

Facing Page: Anna Pavlova and Mikhail Mordkin in the Autumn section of her popular *Bacchanale,* taken from the programme for their visit to Vancouver in 1910, part of an extensive North American tour.

Top: The Misses Sarah and Amy Sternberg were prominent in Toronto dance teaching circles from 1891 to 1930, with Miss Amy taking control of the family studio when her sister married in 1910. This photograph of Miss Amy Sternberg is taken from the programme for her "fantastic extravaganza" at Toronto's Massey Hall in 1915 in aid of the Red Cross Fund. (Courtesy Jean Harper Tilley)

Bottom: Pupils of Miss Amy Sternberg present *The Four Seasons* alfresco in Toronto in the 1920s. (Courtesy Jean Harper Tilley)

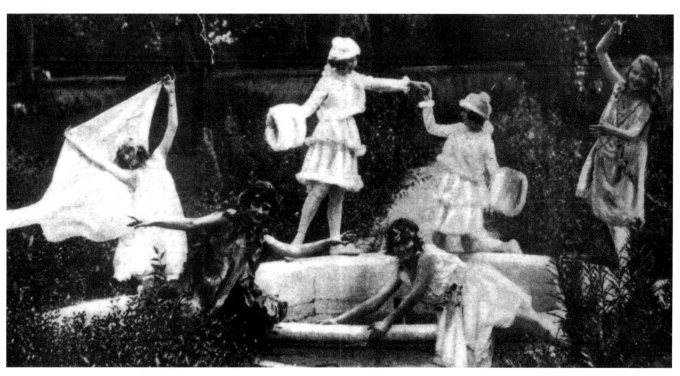

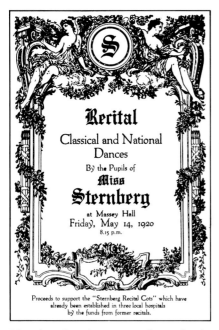

Miss Amy Sternberg's annual recitals of classical and national dances by her pupils were popular events of the 1920s, filling Massey Hall's 2,765 seats on two consecutive nights, proceeds going to support the Sternberg Recital Cots at city hospitals. These photographs of Marjorie Mason (*this page*) and Betty Compton (*facing page*) are taken from magazine montages of the period. Compton went on to do a specialty dance in the New York stage version of *Funny Face* with Fred and Adele Astaire in the late 1920s. (Courtesy Jean Harper Tilley)

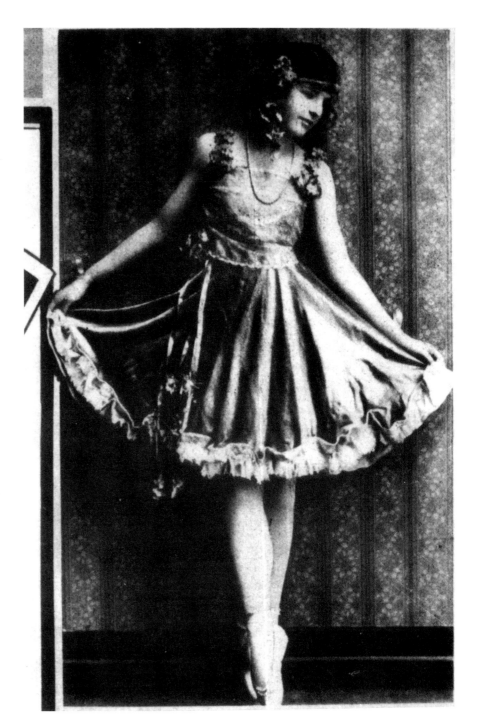

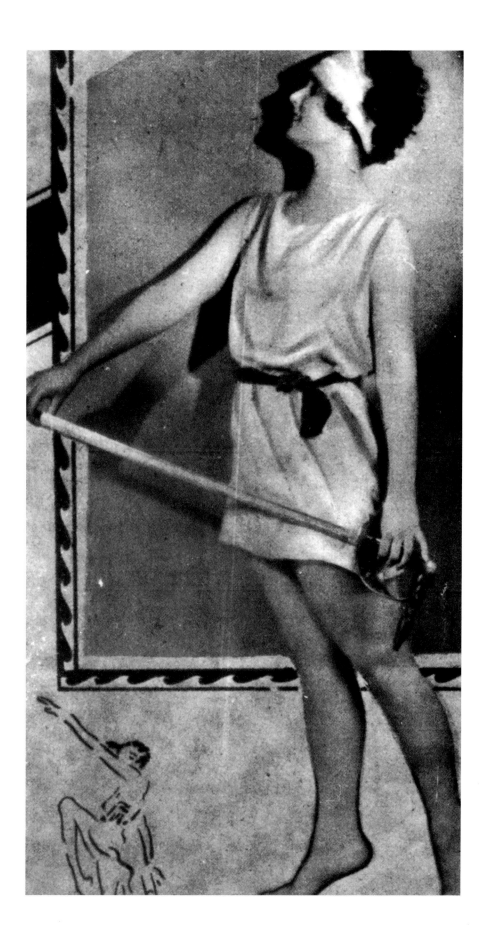

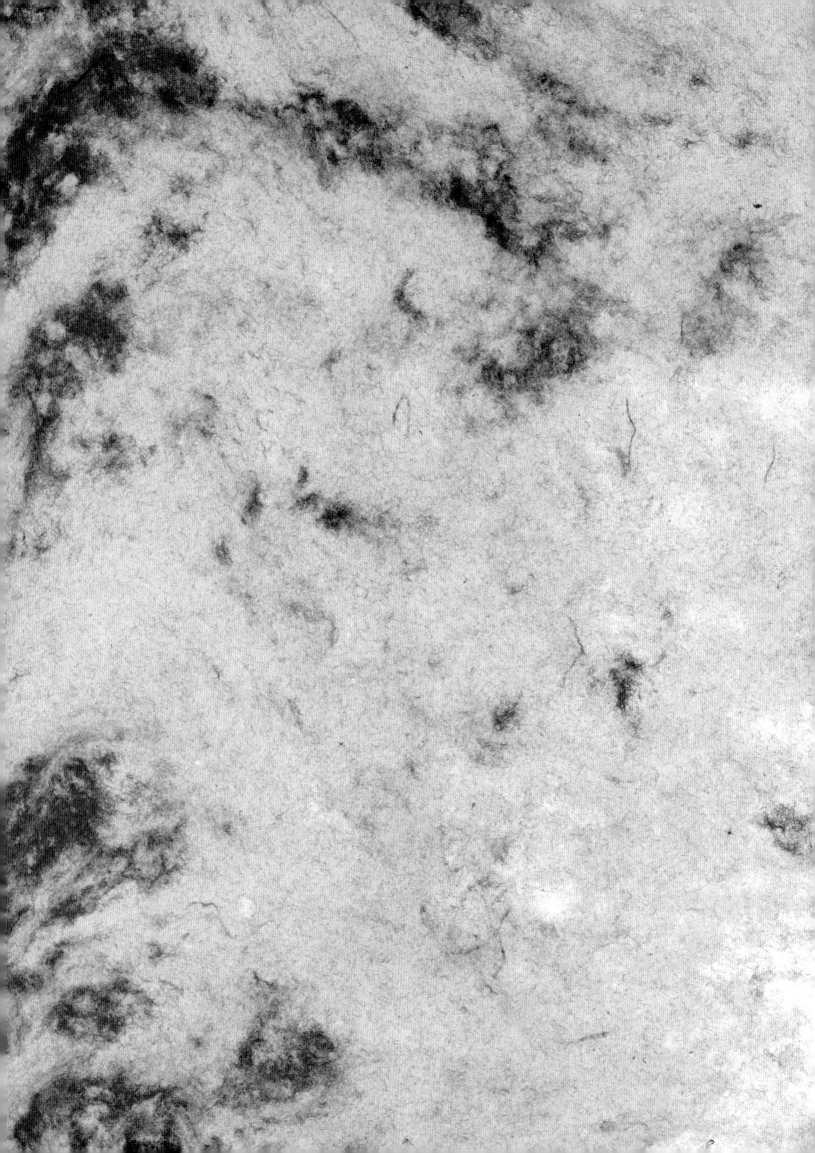

THE EARLY YEARS:

1900–1950

Ballet

INSPIRATION TO DANCE: *The Ballets Russes*

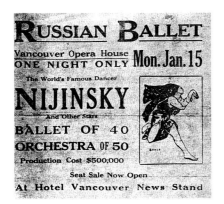

When the Diaghilev Ballets Russes company performed in Vancouver in 1917, with Vaslav Nijinsky as both public draw and acting company head, the Vancouver Daily Sun *reviewer called Diaghilev "the Russian super-Wagner" and commented that "the spectator learns a new and not dangerous discontent with all music that is not also danced and painted, and with all dance or colorist's art which is not also synchronized with orchestra." (*Vancouver Daily Sun *advertisement)*

By the end of the nineteenth century, ballet in Europe was artistically bankrupt. Even in Russia, the form had become sterile and hidebound. At the Maryinsky Theatre in Leningrad, when Michel Fokine (pupil of Petipa, first partner of Pavlova) wanted barefoot dancers for a ballet on a Greek theme, the performers were forced to wear pink tights on which toes had been painted.

But Fokine, one foot in the past and one in the future, knew that there was more to dance than this. Like the pioneering modernist Isadora Duncan, though in entirely different ways, he wanted to give his art a new vitality, a new unity of elements, a new relevance.

It was not a vision that was encouraged at the Maryinsky, and when Fokine was offered the chance to make new ballets for Serge Diaghilev's Ballets Russes company, he leaped at the chance. It was, like Rudolf Nureyev's vault across the airport barrier in Paris more than half a century later, a fateful jump—not merely for the individual, but for the art form. The Diaghilev company's 1909 performances in Paris—with Fokine and his integrationist theories at the choreographic forefront—effectively mark the beginning of modern ballet.

Audiences long resigned to lacklustre performance, dull choreography and uninspiring settings were suddenly dazzled by a savage and exciting modernity. Gweneth Lloyd, who would much later found the Royal Winnipeg Ballet, remembered her first encounter with the Ballets Russes in 1918: "Everything had been pastel before, and suddenly there was all this brilliance."

Diaghilev's influence on North America was initially less pronounced. But over the long term, the company, and the companies it spawned, were to change conceptions of dancing on a stage. In a 1911 Canadian visit, the vaudeville star Gertrude Hoffman was the headliner in a company in which two Diaghilev stars, Lydia Lopokova and Alexandre Volinine, danced part of *Les Sylphides* as a supporting number. Diaghilev's company made its only Canadian appearance, in Vancouver in 1917, with Nijinsky's *Bluebird, Prince Igor*, and Flora Revalles in *Cléopâtre*.

Serge Lifar, a former Diaghilev principal danced with *his* Russian Ballet in Canada in 1933. And that January, Michel Fokine gave his last public performance in Toronto, during a two-week visit to conduct a teaching course at the Russian Ballet School of Dimitri Vladimiroff. Jean Tilley, who attended the Fokine course, found him "a perfectionist, demanding yet understanding." The Vladimiroffs gave a farewell party for Fokine and his wife Vera, and for the singers of the Don Cossack Chorus, who were at Massey Hall the same week. "At dawn the party broke up," Tilley recalled. "We staggered down the stairs . . . accompanied by the heavenly voices of the Cossack choir. It was a sad but glorious farewell."

The de Basil Ballet Russe company made its Canadian debut in Toronto in the fall of 1934. In a perceptive analysis for *Saturday Night*, Lucy Van Gogh suggested it embodied elements of both the original Russian ballet of the imperial opera-houses, and Russian vaudeville, and commented: "The resultant artform is considerably less serious than the ballet from which it is derived. But it retains great qualities of poetic imagination and terpsichorean skill, and adds to them a much broader sense of comic pantomime, producing an entertainment which is admirably suited for North American audiences." Léonide Massine's spectacular and theatrical specialties for the company—symphonic visualizations and character ballets—dictated North American tastes in ballet for close to a decade.

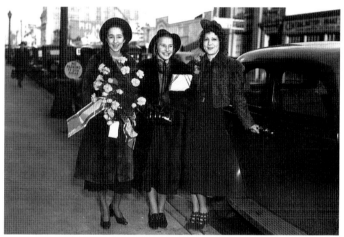

Vancouver, February 3, 1938, close to midnight. Three young ballet students wait nervously for an audition. The de Basil Ballet Russe company is in town, and ballet-master David Lichine has been persuaded by teacher June Roper to take a look at the cream of her student crop.

The children have been trained well, and their tension falls away as they dance everything they know, including tricks like double and triple turns and fouettés. *At the end of two hours, de Basil tells June Roper: "Never before have I seen such excellent training. Madame, I take my hat off to you."*

Patricia Meyers, who is 15, and Rosemary Deveson, who is 16, are offered contracts. Four days later, they join the company on tour, at Portland, Oregon. Rosemary Sankey, taller than the average ballerina of the day, is turned down, though within the year she will be working in Broadway musicals under the name of Maria de Galanta.

Rosemary Deveson and Patricia Meyers with June Roper, as the girls prepare to leave Vancouver to take up their new positions as members of the de Basil Ballet Russe company, February 1938. (Courtesy Leland Windreich)

Born in Rosebud, Texas, June Roper was inspired to dance, like so many others, by Pavlova's example. Her greatest influence was the Los Angeles teacher Ernest Belcher, father of Broadway and Hollywood dancing star Marge Champion. He stressed the bold theatrical effect—an emphasis that was be an important element of June Roper's own success as a teacher.

At the age of 14 the girl was dancing the Goddess of Love at the Pantages Theatre in Los Angeles and later toured Europe; she stopped performing at the age of 26. She arrived in Vancouver in 1934, to visit her sister. Two society women, Yvonne Firkins and Vivien Ramsay, had decided to set up a theatre school covering all aspects of the performing arts. When they heard that June Roper was in town, they invited her to head the school's dance division.

The de Basil company had made its first Vancouver appearance in February, 1935. Four months after the company's visit, June Roper presented the first of a series of school recitals she called Stars of Tomorrow. No title could have been more apt. Her career as a teacher lasted only five years, but in those five years she turned out over 60 professional dancers. June Roper's career as what *Dance-Magazine* would later term "North America's greatest star-maker" had begun.

Pat Meyers (known as Alexandra Denisova) and Rosemary Deveson (who became Natasha Sobinova) created their first new roles in London in July 1938, in Lichine's *Protée*, a ballet about a sea god, inspired by Lichine's first encounter with the girls in Vancouver. A great future for Meyers was prophesied. However, at the age of 18 she married Alberto Alonso, brother-in-law of the great Cuban dancer Alicia Alonso, and together they took over direction of the principal dance academy in Cuba. In 1944 Alberto Alonso moved to New York, and Denisova made her way to Hollywood where, as Patricia Denise, she became a movie dance captain, working on *Seven Brides for Seven Brothers* and *It's Always Fair Weather*.

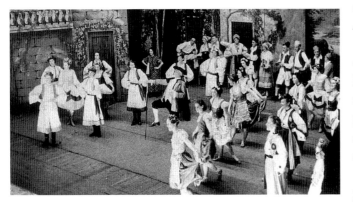

The ensemble from Act I of the first Canadian production of Coppélia, *produced by Dorothy Wilson at the Royal Theatre, Victoria, B.C., 22–23 May 1936. (Victoria Ballet Society photograph, courtesy Leland Windreich)*

Deveson/Sobinova was also warmly welcomed. Lichine created a part for her in *Graduation Ball* (it became one of his most popular works), and London critic Arnold Haskell thought she had the potential to become "a lyrical dancer as personal and unusual as Riabouchinska herself." However, she quit the company in 1941, returned to Vancouver and settled down to teach.

Early in 1939, Sergei Denham's new Ballet Russe company, with Massine as artistic director, appeared in Vancouver, and another Roper student, Ian Gibson, auditioned. Originally trained in Victoria by Dorothy Wilson (who produced North America's first *Coppélia* in Victoria in 1936, with Gibson as Franz), he was accepted by Massine and followed him to Lucia Chase's new Ballet Theatre (later American Ballet Theatre) in New York, dancing several roles originated by Nijinsky. Anton Dolin, describing his dancing in *Le Spectre de la rose*, wrote: "His jump was amazing, and though I never saw Nijinsky dance, I feel sure that Gibson rose as high and as effortlessly into the air, and flew through the window for the final exit as Nijinsky did in those earlier and legendary days." A brilliant career was anticipated, but shortly after taking on the role of Eugene Loring's *Billy the Kid* in 1942, Gibson enlisted in the Canadian Navy, and his wartime duties took such a toll on his health that he never returned to dancing. Had he done so he would almost certainly have become the first *danseur noble* produced in Canada.

Joy Darwin went to the Ballet Jooss in 1937, after refusing a year's free study at the Martha Graham school because she didn't like the prospect of having to minimize her facial expressiveness. Margaret Banks left the Roper school in 1939 for Sadler's Wells; the following year, Jean Hunt (as Kira Bounina) went to de Basil's Original Ballet Russe, and Audree Thomas, as Anna Istomina, to Massine's company. Soon, Roper dancers were being accepted without audition. In 1941, Duncan Noble (actually Duncan Noble MacGillivray) went to Ballet Theatre on the word of June Roper alone—she wired Massine to say she had another boy ready, and a contract came by return from Lucia Chase. The same year, Robert Lindgren was accepted by the Denham Ballet Russe, but the War Manpower Commission refused him permission to work with the company, and he had to wait for an invitation from Massine to join Ballet Theatre in 1943 before his professional dance career could begin. He later became prominent as a dance academic in the United States.

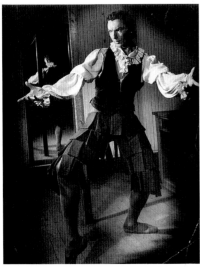

Duncan Noble, another June Roper alumnus, danced with Ballet Theatre and the Ballet Russe de Monte Carlo. He appears here in the revised 1949 Ballet Russe production of Antonia Cobos's The Mute Wife. *(Will Rapport photograph, courtesy Leland Windreich)*

Peggy Middleton gave up her ambition to be an opera singer for a career in the movies—under the name of Yvonne de Carlo. And other Roper dancers found work at New York's Radio City Music Hall, on Broadway and in nightclubs.

June Roper was not the first teacher in Canada to send dancers to the international companies of Europe and New York. At the beginning of the 1930s, Ottawa's Gwendolyn Osborne, a Boston-born teacher of ballet and Duncan-style interpretive movement, sent her pupil Nesta Williams to Europe, where she danced in London and with the short-lived Ballet Russe de Paris (under Margaret Severn, a mask specialist who later retired to Vancouver) before joining the Ballet Russe de Monte Carlo. She married company dancer Sviatoslav Toumine and as Nesta Toumine eventually settled in Ottawa.

The sisters Nora and Patricia White also both took their initial training with Gwendolyn Osborne in the late 1930s. Nora, the elder, left first for studies in New York, later graduating to the Denham Ballet Russe. Patricia followed, as Patricia Wilde, in 1945, at the age of 17, making her professional debut two years later in the Marquis de Cuevas's Ballet International. In 1950 she launched a 15-year career as a star of George Balanchine's New York City Ballet.

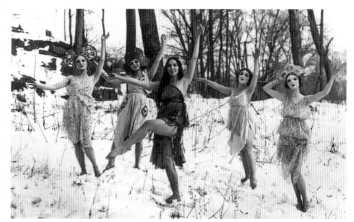

Mask specialist Margaret Severn, photographed in New York in the 1920s. She eventually settled in Vancouver. (Courtesy Margaret Severn)

Montreal sent Robert Bell to the de Basil company in 1935 (he became Boris Belsky, stayed until 1941, and returned as *régisseur* in 1947). In the same period, another Montreal dancer, Emmy Sharples (Russianized into Kira Sharova), was with de Basil's company; in 1941 she danced in her home town on the company's last visit.

Few of the dancers who left Canada returned.

———

Many of the individuals prominent in the early development of professional theatrical dancing in Canada were also pioneers in dance education. Most teachers dabbled in amateur production as an offshoot of their studio activities. In Toronto, a prominent teacher in the early decades of the century was Samuel Titchener-Smith, who sent a number of students to professional careers abroad.

In Montreal, one of the best-regarded was Mary Beetles, an Englishwoman who taught at George W. Shefler's studio before opening her own school in 1931. Among the ballets she presented was a version of *Les Sylphides.* One of Shefler's students, Micheline Petolas, went on to a career in New York and Hollywood.

Maurice Morenoff (Morenoff was a professional name—the family name was Lacasse) taught in Montreal from about 1931, continuing a business established by his father before the turn of the century. He choreographed for religious pageants, operettas and his "ballet music-hall" troupe—a company whose emphasis was more ballet than music-hall, using light classical music as the basis for free ballet interpretations. Though amateur, it was regarded for years as the principal performing ensemble in and about the city. Other contributors to the teaching mix in Montreal in the late 1920s to 1940s included Isak Ruvenoff, a temperamental and gregarious Russian émigré who taught the German Zorn method, stressing a gruelling barre and a strong adage. And Tatiana Lipkovska, a former Kirov student and member of the de Basil company, settled in the city with her husband,

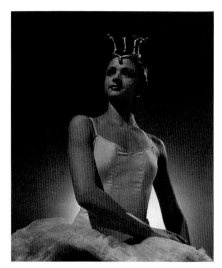

In 1942 Boris Volkoff invited Dance News *editor Anatole Chujoy to provide a candid private assessment of his company. Chujoy picked out Mildred Herman (later Melissa Hayden) as the one female with potential to become "a great ballerina." Volkoff thought her such an odd choice he never bothered to tell her of Chujoy's praise. (Ronny Jaques photograph, courtesy Ruth Carse)*

the impresario Nicolas Koudriavtzeff, and opened a successful school.

Russianness held similar sway on the West Coast. In Vancouver, Nikolas Merinoff shared a studio with Charlotte del Roy, and Boris Novikoff had studios with his sister, Tatiana Platowa. Born in 1897 in Kazan, Novikoff fled with his family after the Revolution and arrived in Vancouver in the 1920s. According to his privately published memoirs, he set up a Russian-American Ballet Company, and performed extensively around Vancouver and in Victoria. He and his brother Ivan (who had settled in Seattle) took a company of four on a West Coast tour under the title Ballet Bureau, Inc. Shortly thereafter he and his sister moved to the U.S.

In Victoria, meanwhile, Nicholas Rusanoff, who claimed to have been with the Imperial Russian Ballet in Moscow, joined forces in the late 1920s with Dorothy Wilson, who had moved to Victoria from England in 1922 and with her daughter Doreen had established a dance school in a church basement. The advertisement for the opening of their Russian Ballet School of Dancing in 1927 covered all the angles—"Limbering, Stretching, Ballet, Classical, Interpretive, Toe, Character, Adagio, Stage, Acrobatic, the Black Bottom and All Types."

———

Boris Volkoff, the man who prepared the way for the eventual creation of the National Ballet of Canada, was, so the legend goes, smuggled into Canada by a pair of hired thugs.

Born Boris Baskakoff into a farming family near Moscow in 1900 or 1902, he studied at the state ballet school in Moscow and danced with the Mordkin Ballet. On tour in Siberia, he skipped the company and fled to Shanghai, where he joined the obscure Stavrinsky Ballet Russe for a tour of Southeast Asia. According to Volkoff, Hong Kong audiences had not seen ballet for years and welcomed the company enthusiastically. Unfortunately, the pre-performance hospitality was excessive: as the curtain went up on the opening number, *Bacchus*, the orchestra broke into the music for *Schéhérazade* and the cast burst enthusiastically onto the stage wearing costumes for *Prince Igor*.

When the troupe was disbanded, Volkoff made his way to Chicago: rather than be deported, he opted to make a dash to Canada. According to his former wife, the dancer and teacher Janet Baldwin, Volkoff (or a friend) "hired two thugs, and they stuck a big cigar in Boris's mouth and told him to shut up and let them do the talking, and they drove him across the border."

His arrival in Toronto was opportune. Leon Leonidoff and Florence Rogge, Toronto's leading dancer-choreographers, had just left for New York, where she choreographed and produced at Radio City Music Hall for a decade. Their departure left a vacancy for a lead dancer and ballet master in the live *divertissements* presented between films at the Loew's Uptown movie house. Almost immediately, Volkoff found himself dancing *Jardin de plaisir* with the Uptown Girls.

By 1931, the Boris Volkoff School of Dancing was offering regular public recitals, featuring Volkoff doing a "dramatic interpretation" of, say, a Chopin polonaise, and his students performing, typically, *Caucasian Sketches* and *Holiday in Russia*. He was a short, snarling man, volatile and unpredictable, fond of striking insouciant and worldly poses, rarely without his ivory cigarette holder and his little cap. "He played the role of the teacher-tyrant—the Hollywood-typecast dancemaster," recalled former student Duncan Cameron. "He adored the girls, he really did care about them, but he was terribly frustrated that no one was interested in dancing."

Some of them were. Mildred Herman, who as Melissa Hayden spent almost a quarter-century as a principal with the New York City Ballet, took her first classes with Volkoff. She remembers him (in her book, *Dancer to Dancer*) as "a wonderful teacher who was consistent and exact, who never confused me, who never made dance boring but always a challenge."

Volkoff's first professional breakthrough was an engagement to choreograph a ballet for the annual carnival of the Toronto Skating Club in 1933. He couldn't stand up on skates himself, so at rehearsal he would rush around with a cushion tied to his seat, and canvas overboots on his feet. Volkoff always claimed to have been the inventor of the ice ballet; he was certainly one of the first to create full-scale ice choreographies of *Swan Lake* and *Prince Igor*.

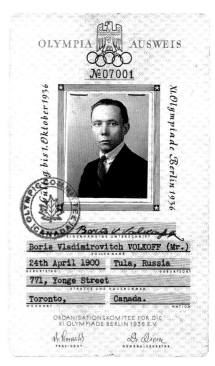

His dancers were not paid, and their technical prowess was limited; by day, they worked in garages, shops, factories and colleges. But they were filled with enthusiasm and ambition. In 1936 he took a group of them to dance as Canada's official representatives at the International Tanzwettspiele, part of Hitler's Summer Olympics in Berlin. The programme contained two of the earliest examples of original dancework created on Canadian themes to Canadian music—*Mala*, an Eskimo legend about a shaman's journey, to music by Sir Ernest MacMillan based on Indian chant; and *Mon-Ka-Ta*, which used masks and totems derived from West Coast Indian designs, performed to music of Bartok, Satie and Indian folk tunes arranged by Marius Barbeau.

Volkoff's group was one of five chosen for honourable mention at the end of the noncompetitive festivities. The accolade won him new respect in Canada.

Hopeful and excited, he wanted the logical next step. "Canada could and should have a repertory ballet company," he wrote in *Curtain Call* magazine in the fall of 1938, and in May 1939, at Massey Hall, Toronto, he made a serious attempt to launch one—the Boris Volkoff Ballet Company. The programme also called it the First Canadian Ballet; it was an unpaid ensemble of 20 women and 10 men, and they danced six ballets. Toronto *Star* critic Augustus Bridle was ecstatic. "Canada now has the germ of a national ballet," he wrote, "with Toronto as its logical birthplace."

Artistic director's pass issued to Boris Volkoff for the 1936 Olympic Games in Berlin. Volkoff's ensemble was one of 26 groups (including the modernist companies of Mary Wigman and Harald Kreutzberg) participating in the International Tanzwettspiele. (Courtesy Janet Baldwin)

A PRAIRIE FLOWER: The Royal Winnipeg Ballet

Winnipeg, summer, 1937. Gweneth Lloyd, an English dance teacher, is in the city to visit a friend who has moved to Canada from England some years before.

Pausing for rest in a city park while out walking, Gweneth asks a woman who is sharing her bench about the state of ballet on the prairies.

"Ballet?" says the woman. "I've never heard of it." To Gweneth, that sounds like a challenge, and a challenge is just what she needs to hear.

Excited by what she considers the city's possibilities for growth, she hurries back to England to recruit the assistance of a colleague. They set sail for their new home late the following spring.

———

The early development of ballet in Canada was deeply rooted not only in the Russian but in the British ballet tradition—itself derived, in part at least, from the Diaghilev legacy. That legacy had been carried to Britain by two women—Marie Rambert, born Miriam Rambam or Ramberg in Poland in 1888, and Ninette de Valois, born Edris Stannus in Ireland in 1898.

Rambert, trained in eurhythmics by the system's originator, Emile Jacques Dalcroze, taught the method to Diaghilev's Ballets Russes. She later opened a school in London that developed into Britain's first permanent company, the Ballet Rambert.

Ninette de Valois trained in London, joined the Diaghilev company in 1923, and later also opened a ballet school in London. In 1931, in association with Lilian Baylis of the Old Vic Theatre, she established the Vic-Wells Ballet, later renamed the Sadler's Wells—the direct forerunner of today's Royal Ballet.

Rambert and de Valois were not the first to introduce ballet as a serious art in England. Adeline Genée, born Anina Jensen in Denmark in 1878, was founder-president at the 1920 launching of the Association of Operatic Dancing—an institution that today, as the Royal Academy of Dancing (RAD), maintains strict standards of academic classical dance, conducting examinations in many countries, including Canada.

Canada's first and for a time only recorded member of the RAD was Dorothy Cox, who ran a school in London, Ontario. But it was not until the arrival in Winnipeg of Gweneth Lloyd and Betty Farrally in 1938, and the return to Canada of London-trained, Toronto-born Bettina Byers the following year, that the codified teaching and examination systems of the RAD began to establish a foothold. Byers was the first RAD organizer in Canada; in 1946 Mara McBirney, an Englishwoman, settled in Vancouver, where she taught for many years, adjudicated for the RAD and directed, either alone or with others, a succession of amateur ballet troupes.

———

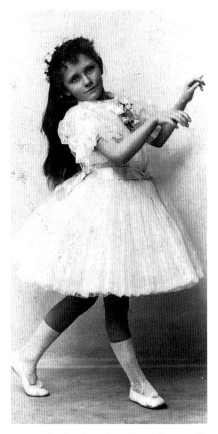

Gweneth Lloyd, co-founder of the Royal Winnipeg Ballet, aged five or six, posed in Cambridge, England, by her grandmother, who instructed the child to "Make your hands look pretty, dear!" (Courtesy Gweneth Lloyd)

The fact that Gweneth Lloyd and Betty Farrally left England for Winnipeg was purely accidental. The fact that they would go on to lay the foundations of what is now the second-oldest ballet company in North America, and one of the world's most-travelled, is a fortuity of history.

Gweneth Lloyd was born in Eccles, near Manchester, in 1901. She began her career as a teacher of gymnastics and did not develop a serious interest in dance until she came into contact in the mid-1920s with what was known then as natural movement, based on ancient Greek dance forms. She supplemented these studies with tuition in a variety of other dance forms, and in 1927 opened the Torch School of Dancing in Leeds, Yorkshire.

Betty Hey (she became Betty Farrally in 1942) was enrolled at the Torch school in 1932, when she was 17, and later joined Gweneth on the Torch staff.

The two women hit Winnipeg like summertime whirlwinds—such energy, such style—and within months had established not only a teaching business but, for their advanced students, the Winnipeg Ballet Club.

In 1939 they were asked to provide two pieces of dance on prairie themes for a pageant celebrating a visit to the city by George VI and Queen Elizabeth—"about five minutes each," said the alderman in charge, "and plenty of leg." They were Gweneth Lloyd's first attempts at choreography—*Grain*, a mimetic piece about the wheat cycle, and *Kilowatt Magic*, all whirling arms and rattling cellophane to signify the coming of hydro-electric power to the prairie: perhaps the earliest examples in Canada of social-issue dance, and effectively the public debut of the Royal Winnipeg Ballet.

With the assistance of a trio of enthusiasts from three significant strata of Winnipeg life—Lady Madge Tupper, wife of a prominent lawyer and a ferocious advocate of the arts; John Russell, dean of architecture at the University of Manitoba and a designer for amateur theatricals; and David Yeddeau, a veteran of all aspects of theatrical production—the club flourished, and by June 1940, Gweneth felt confident enough to present its first full-scale performance.

Her principles of programming emphasized the art's accessibility. "Ballet," she said, "is no longer a champagne and caviar treat, ballet is a beer and skittles entertainment." Like Diaghilev before her, she built triple-bill programmes that offered something for everyone—typically, in Winnipeg, a romantic white ballet for the ladies, a comic ballet for the reluctant husbands, and something in a modern vein for those who liked to think. The first programme defined the format—*Divertissements* in the classical manner, to music of Arensky; a three-act comedy ballet called *The Wager*; and an expanded version of *Kilowatt Magic*. From the start, the Winnipeg Ballet was a company for the ordinary dancegoer; and ordinary dancegoers the world over have warmed to that.

The company for that first performance was a motley crew—stenographers, teachers, clerks, a figure-skating champion, a carpenter, a competition diver—but it also contained the seeds of the company's first starring roster: Paddy Stone, then 16, later to build a successful career as a variety choreographer in England—and to return to Winnipeg to give the company two of its all-time best-selling ballets, *Variations on Strike Up the Band* and *The Hands*; Jean McKenzie, the company's first female lead and later the founding principal of the company school; and a shy nine-year-old called David Adams, who would go on to a distinguished career in ballet in Canada and London.

The young company found financial shelter under the wing of the Richardson family, influential in the development of Winnipeg life since the start of the twentieth century. Muriel Sprague Richardson donated generously, helping to raise funds and freely contributing business guidance and artistic advice. After 1955 the responsibility was assumed by her daughter Kathleen, an early participant in Gweneth Lloyd's Greek dance classes.

Despite its financial shakiness, the company made steady artistic progress. In 1943 an editorial writer was convinced the company was "on its shining way to greatness."

In the audience during a visit by the Ballet Russe de Monte Carlo to the Walker Theatre in 1942 was the individual who would, many years later, lead the company on that shining way, Arnold Spohr. A lanky, sensitive musician and sports enthusiast, he had been dragged to the theatre by his sister because no one else would

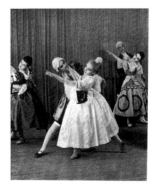

The WINNIPEG BALLET CLUB

presents

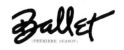

(PREMIERE SEASON)

PLAYHOUSE THEATRE
JUNE 11 and 12 *1939*   8.45 P.M.

VERY PRECIOUS

Gweneth Lloyd inscribed the words "Very Precious" on her own souvenir copy of the programme for the Winnipeg Ballet Club's first full public performance, in 1940— though she dated it a year early. (Courtesy Gweneth Lloyd)

take her. It was his first experience of ballet—Massine, Tamara Toumanova, Frederic Franklin, all of them spouting personality and emotion—and it was a revelation. "I was in another world," he recalled much later. "It was magic."

With the exception of a single work by Paddy Stone, the entire repertoire for the company's first decade was created by Lloyd. She made three or four ballets a year, each built to suit the dancing talents she was working with and to take best advantage of her own skills. She was particularly good at programming that drew inspiration from the work of the touring companies. Léonide Massine's *Les Présages*, for instance, was a model for Gweneth's *Les Préludes*—in her own words, "The same type of thing, all very symbolic-cum-abstract-cum Dali!!"

The ballet classics were her weak point—she had never been a professional performer—and she stayed well clear of the better-known staples. It was not until David Adams returned from a London jaunt in 1948, bearing such choreographic spoils as Nijinsky's *Le Spectre de la rose* and extracts from London's versions of *Swan Lake* and *The Sleeping Beauty*, that the Winnipeggers began to give their audiences homemade versions of the classical repertoire.

Instead, the Winnipeg Ballet—unable to survive by performances in Winnipeg alone, and therefore forced to tour—defined itself very early in its professional career as a small, highly portable contemporary ballet company.

SHARED DREAMS: The Ballet Festivals

It is an irony of history that it was a joint initiative of the Winnipeg group and Boris Volkoff—either of which might reasonably have been thought at the time to be prime candidates to run a national ballet company—that was to lead to the creation of the National Ballet of Canada.

The demands of war had depleted Volkoff's performing ranks, but not his ambitions, and his determination won him admiration. "Mr. Volkoff has made a brave and extremely promising start," wrote Robertson Davies in *Saturday Night* in May 1941. "It is to be hoped that his work will not be brought to nothing by lack of public support. Canadians, being a sensible and artistic people (though they may deny the latter charge hotly) are fond of ballet; here is a chance for them to acquire one of their own."

Anatole Chujoy, editor of New York's *Dance News*, added his voice to the general cry for a national company for Canada, but it was Paul Duval, in *Saturday Night* in November 1945, who capped articulate reasons for the creation of a Diaghilev-style company with practical suggestions as to how to make it happen.

"No other art form except opera can express the richness of a nation's composite arts so completely as ballet," he wrote. "We have in Canada painters capable of creating first-rate decors and costumes . . . what a variety of designs Fritz Brandtner, Lawren Harris, Alfred Pellan and Paul-Emile Borduas might produce! Native English and French composers like Healey Willan, Geoffrey Ridout and Robert Farnum [*sic*] to name only three are fully equipped to write native ballet suites. And as for native themes, French Canada alone—a subject which, so far as I know, has never been treated in ballet—could supply dozens of fruitful ideas." The problem, he said, was that no city in Canada was capable of supporting a permanent company of its own, even with the aid of wealthy sponsors. So what he suggested was the establishment of a touring company based in Ottawa (which was central, and "would also forestall Montreal-Toronto feuding"). Meanwhile, he said, what was needed was a Canadian ballet conference at which anyone interested could exchange views and take stock of needs.

It was on its way—but not in Toronto, or Montreal or even in neutral Ottawa. In Winnipeg.

———

In March 1947, the Winnipeg Ballet and the Boris Volkoff company were invited to take part in an international choreographic competition in Copenhagen. The two groups barely knew the other existed. Both asked for support from Ottawa to appear as representatives of Canada at the contest, and both were turned down. Later, at a party in Toronto, David Yeddeau, manager of the Winnipeg Ballet, met Volkoff and his wife, Janet Baldwin. Struck by the fact that the two groups had been able to exist for so long with no knowledge of each other, Yeddeau suggested a dance festival to spread the word about dance's blossoming.

Yeddeau subsequently claimed to have written to over 100 ballet schools across Canada, though he was eventually able to find only two other groups who would agree to take part in the festival—Ruth Sorel's modernist company in Montreal, and a group operated by the Vancouver Ballet Society.

Even so: four companies . . . it was a beginning.

An unexpected boost came from Rideau Hall, in Ottawa. The new governor-general, Viscount Alexander of Tunis, was about to make his first trip to western Canada, along with Viscountess Alexander, and an aide called to ask if the vice-regal couple might attend the festival's opening performance. Startled and delighted, Yeddeau and his colleagues made the couple guests of honour.

Three days before the April 29 opening of the festival, the Red River flooded the centre of the city and rendered the original venue unusable. Yeddeau was forced to rescind the invitation to the Vancouver company in order to be able to use the money to offset the higher rental costs of another theatre.

There is a certain neatness about the first festival's final participant list. The event brought together, for the first time, the three principal threads of influence on the early development of dance in Canada: the Russian classical tradition, via Volkoff; modern German expressionism, via Sorel; and early English, via Lloyd.

It was, of necessity, a modest affair. But it was a crucial moment in the story of dance in Canada, because it pushed closer to reality what had until that time been not much more than a shared dream . . . the creation of a National Ballet for Canada.

But not quite yet.

———

Financially, the 1948 ballet festival was a disaster. But it caught the mood of the time.

"This festival has proved that there is enough talent . . . to justify pressing forward to the creation of a Canadian ballet," wrote Randolph Patton in a summing-up in the Winnipeg *Tribune*. "Most essential of all," he wrote, "the forward movement implies that the Canadian people themselves will keep abreast of stirring events, becoming more critical and more responsive—and thereby getting more out of life than is possible on the lukewarm leftovers of other cultures."

An unwillingness to settle for the lukewarm leftovers of other cultures was characteristic of the times. In 1944 the government had set up a committee to study the potential social changes of the postwar era, and 15 arts organizations had marched on Ottawa to convince that committee of the need for a new deal for the the arts. In 1948 the Royal Commission on National Development in the Arts, Letters and Sciences (commonly known as the Massey Commission) was established.

The driving forces behind the first Canadian Ballet Festival, in Winnipeg, 1948 (left to right): Ruth Sorel, David Yeddeau, Gweneth Lloyd and Boris Volkoff. (National Film Board photograph, courtesy Metropolitan Toronto Library)

It was a period of unprecedented popularity for dance in Canada. The country's dance schools had an estimated total enrolment of 15,000 pupils, and when the Sadler's Wells company returned to Toronto in 1951, 80,000 letters were received asking for tickets. Dance even began to influence women's fashions. Ballet slippers became, for a time, the fashionable footwear, and fashion-plate models struck vaguely balletic poses. "Things are going so well," enthused one magazine writer early in 1949, "that there is even some talk that they might start paying the dancers in this country."

The Red Shoes, an English movie about the Diaghilev era, caught the imagination of a generation. Its release in 1948 cleared the way for the Sadler's Wells Ballet's total triumph in North America the following year. According to S. Morgan-Powell in the Montreal *Star*, the company's visit to Canada was "perhaps the most important event of our theatrical story in the past half-century." It was important because it opened people's eyes. The Ballets Russes companies had been popular art in the widest sense, but no one pretended the things they did were subtle or polished; they were bravura exercises in projection, personality and theatricality, with the emphasis on brilliance and entertainment.

Sadler's Wells had the brilliance, but it had style and depth as well. In Canada, as everywhere, the natives were delighted, and eventually that delight turned to envy, and eventually that envy begat the National Ballet of Canada.

But, again, not quite yet.

———

The second Canadian Ballet Festival was held in Toronto in March 1949. Ten companies and 200 dancers participated, representing cities from Vancouver to Montreal, and the five days of performances drew a total audience of 8,400, generating a financial surplus.

One of the festival's most immediate consequences was the stimulation of new Canadian art works through the interaction of artists of different disciplines. Two works on the opening programme used commissioned scores by Canadian composers—Gweneth Lloyd's *Visages*, an allegorical Pilgrim's Progress with masks, to music of Walter Kaufmann; and Ruth Sorel's *La Gaspésienne*, using music of Pierre Brabant. On the second night, Boris Volkoff presented *The Red Ear of Corn*, a setting of an Indian legend, for which he had commissioned the first major score by John Weinzweig.

In his wrap-up piece for the *Globe and Mail*, Anatole Chujoy described the event as "a huge success" and added: "It could be that my interest in the festival was not without a touch of envy. We, in the United States, have yet to plan anything like the Canadian Ballet Festival, and it now seems overdue." He was to persist with this theme. And in 1956, two years after the Canadian ballet festival movement had run its course in Canada and been discarded, Chujoy's urgings finally bore fruit and the U.S. regional ballet festival network was born.

The companies involved in the first two ballet festivals were not, in fact, the only companies active in Canada at the time.

In Ottawa, Nesta Toumine, back from the Ballet Russe, had joined forces with Yolande Leduc to set up a school, out of which was launched the Ottawa Ballet Company. Its first programme, in March 1947, featured the performance debuts of New York–trained Svetlana Beriosova and Nicholas Polajenko, both sub-
sequently to win fame in England and Europe. The programme featured what Toumine claimed was the first staging of *The Nutcracker* in North America. A year later, the company offered what was called the Canadian premiere of *Giselle*—more properly the first Canadian production, since the Russian companies had been presenting *Giselle* in Canada since the mid-1930s. It featured Jean Stoneham, a June Roper pupil from Vancouver, later a principal with the Winnipeg company.

An early attempt to establish ballet in Nova Scotia was the Halifax Ballet, founded by Latvian Jury Gotshalks and his wife Irene Apiné after their immigration to Canada in 1947. And Mildred Wickson in Toronto entered a company from her studio in the 1949 festival.

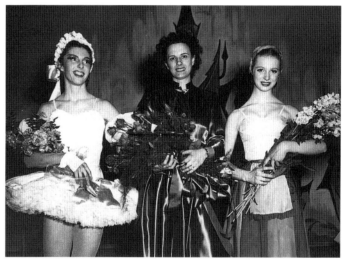

Nesta Toumine broke with Yolande Leduc in 1949 and set up the Ottawa Classical Ballet. She is shown here (centre) *with Joanne Ashe* (left) *and Marilyn Sewell, later with the National Ballet of Canada, after a performance of* Coppélia *that season. (Courtesy Nesta Toumine)*

And although Montreal was only able to muster a single modernist company for the first festival, the city's active dance teaching community, including half a dozen who offered variants on the Russian style, had for two decades mounted modest performances along with the customary school recitals. Early small companies included Paula Dunning's Ballet Metropole, Mary Beetles's Ballet Entre Nous, and Eleanor Moore-Ashton's Montreal Ballet, launched in 1949 and seen at several ballet festivals.

Also in 1949, Gerald Crevier, a pupil of Ruvenoff, an influential teacher and the first RAD organizer in Quebec, founded Les Ballets Quebec. A production in May 1950 was greeted by Brian Macdonald, then writing reviews for the Montreal *Herald*, as "an astonishing reminder of the talent we harbour in our own bosoms." This lavishness of talent may have been its downfall. Four of the company members accepted invitations to join the newly formed National Ballet in 1951, and the following year Crevier closed his school and dissociated himself from dance.

But in terms of the story of dancing in Canada, Montreal's true significance at this time was not in the area of ballet at all.

June Roper in a typical costume for her adagio performances in Europe in the 1920s (*this page*) and as the Goddess of Love in Los Angeles, 1919 (*facing page*). Performing an amalgam of supported adagio, point work, Spanish and popular dance, she became the toast of Europe, sharing bills with Mistinguett and Maurice Chevalier in Paris, and with Jessie Matthews and Tillie Losch in London. (Courtesy Leland Windreich)

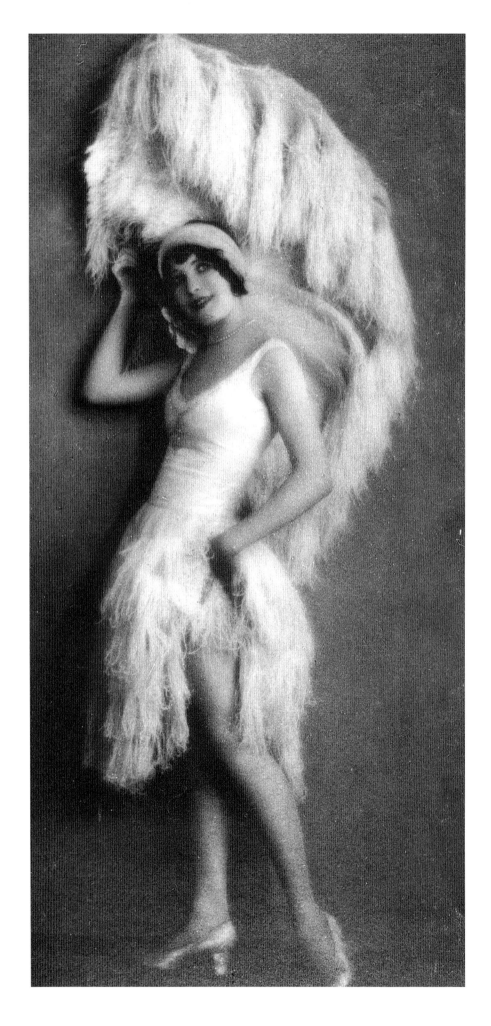

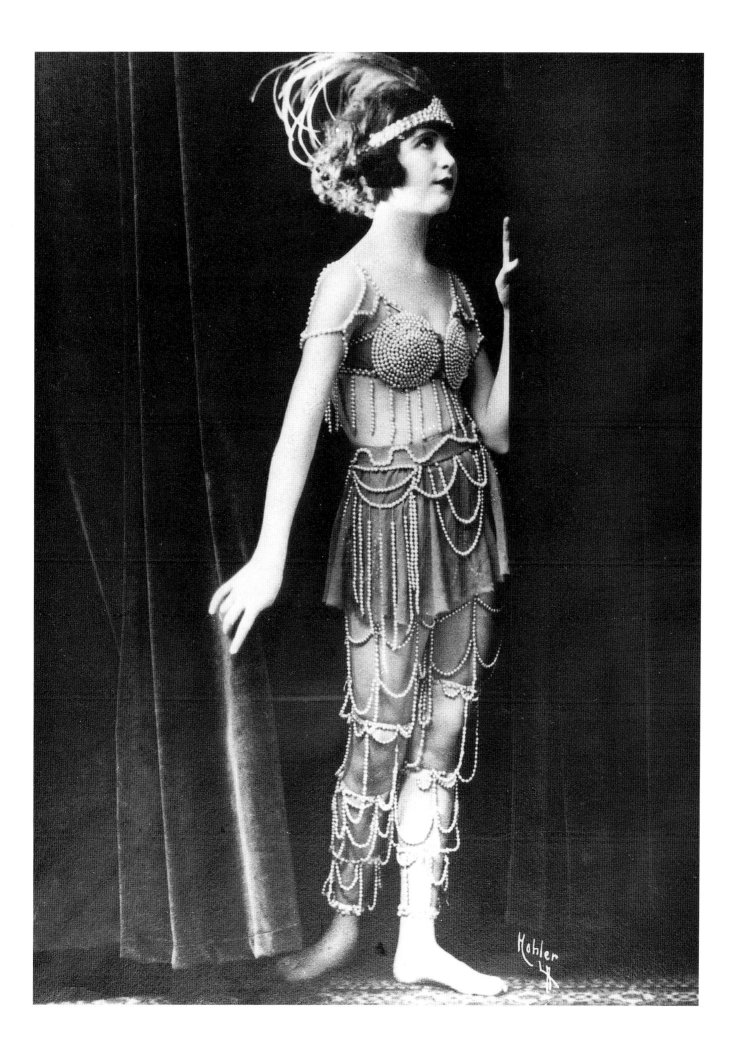

Kohler

Rosemary Deveson (*left*) as the Bird of
Paradise and Joy Darwin as the Fire Bird
in the *Dream Bird Ballet* by June Roper, in
Vancouver in 1936. (Courtesy Leland
Windreich)

Facing page: Rosemary Deveson as the
Bird of Paradise in the *Dream Bird Ballet*
by June Roper. (Courtesy Leland
Windreich)

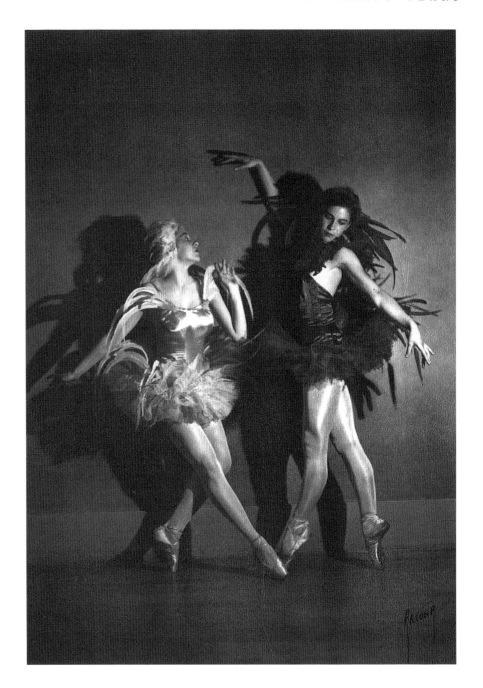

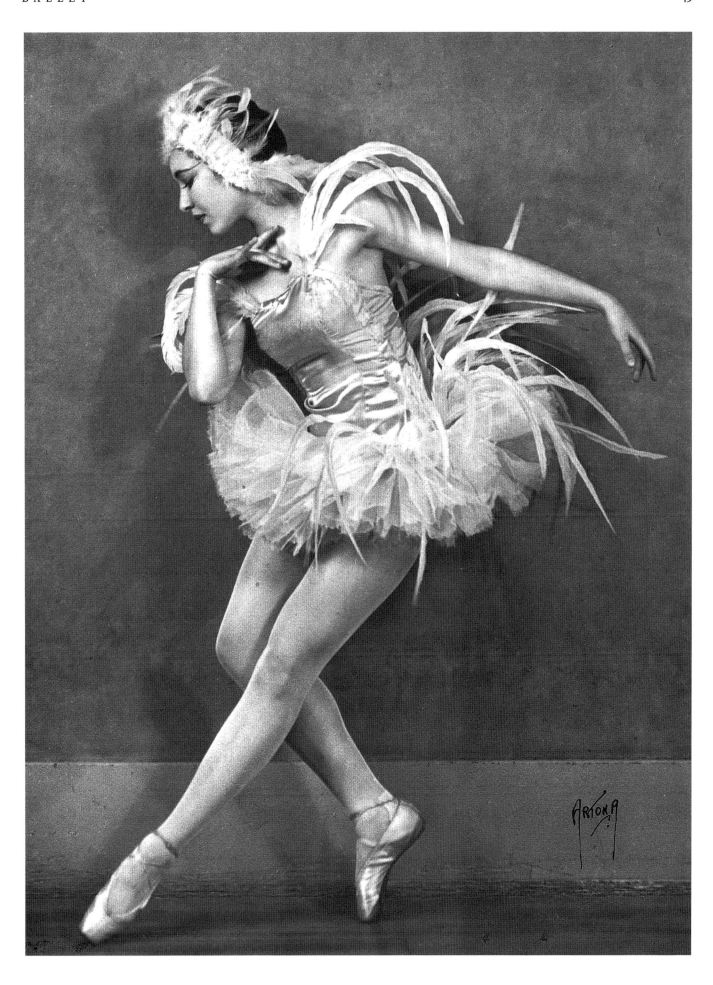

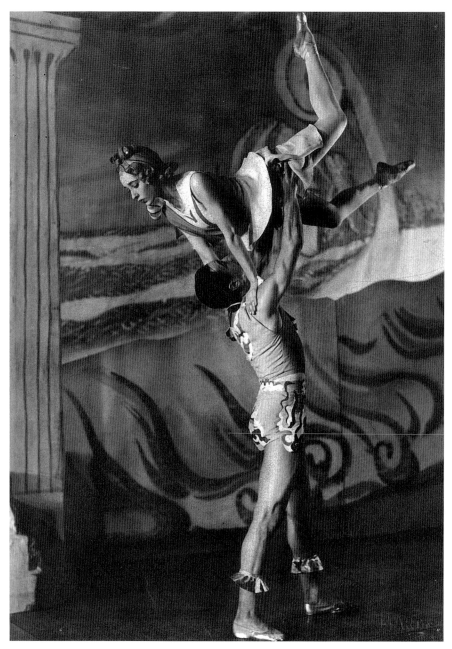

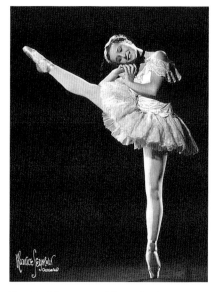

Patricia Meyers, as Alexandra Denisova, in the de Basil Ballet Russe company, 1941. The daughter of a former Tiller Girl in the English music halls, Meyers later called herself Patricia Denise (her middle name) and eventually made a career as a dance captain in Hollywood. (Maurice Seymour photograph, courtesy Leland Windreich)

Facing page: The teenage Ian Gibson demonstrates in Dorothy Wilson's Victoria studio the style that won him a place with Ballet Theatre in New York in the early 1940s. His Bluebird was said to display a technical command "not surpassed and seldom equalled in the contemporary dance theatre." (Courtesy Leland Windreich)

Rosemary Deveson as Natasha Sobinova ("I was named for a Russian tenor I'd never heard of") with David Lichine in his *Protée,* made for Deveson and Patricia Meyers at the de Basil Ballet Russe. (Baron photograph, courtesy Leland Windreich)

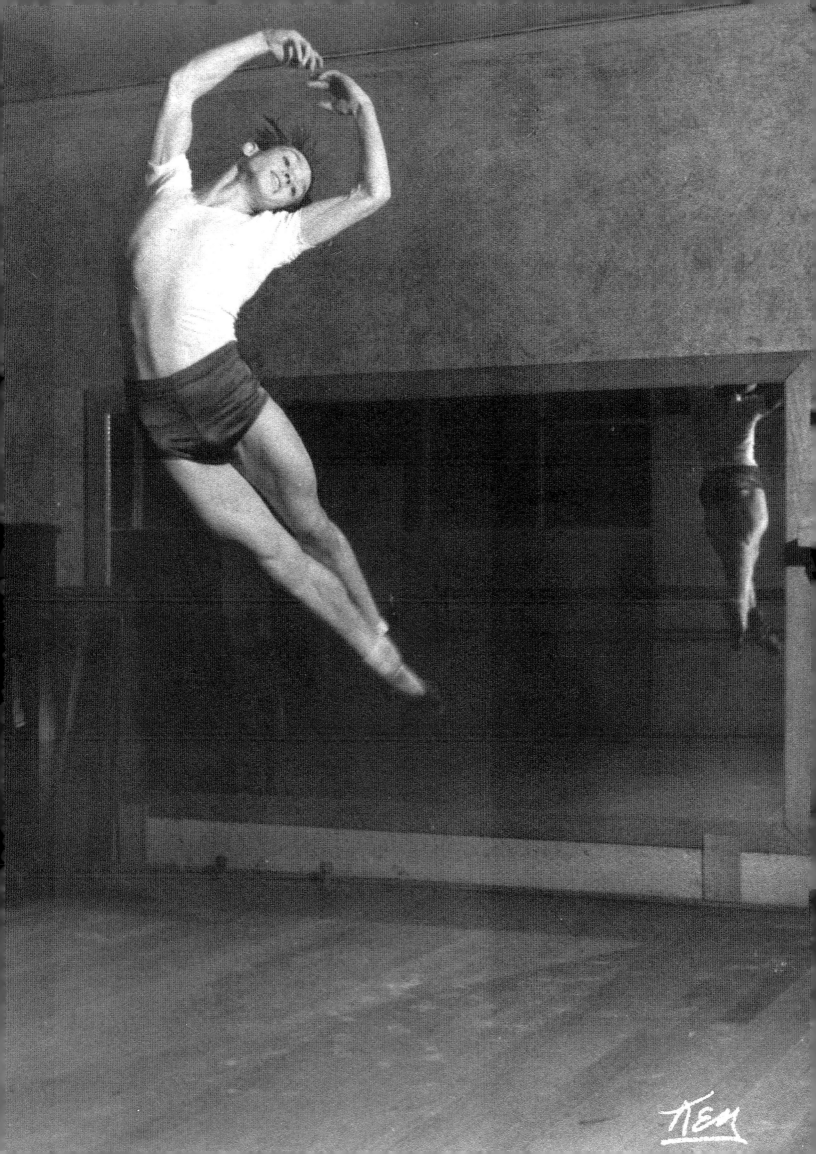

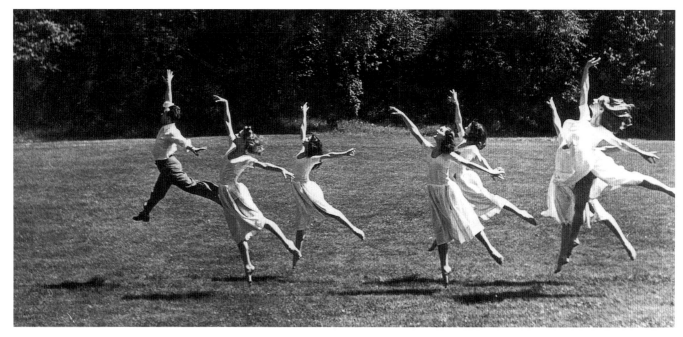

Boris Volkoff leads his dancers across the grass of a Toronto park. The company, said Toronto *Star* critic Augustus Bridle in 1940, "gives leafy June a run for gladness." (Ronny Jaques photograph, courtesy Metropolitan Toronto Library)

Facing page: Boris Volkoff at the barre with student Mildred Herman, who as Melissa Hayden became a principal dancer with the New York City Ballet. (Courtesy Metropolitan Toronto Library)

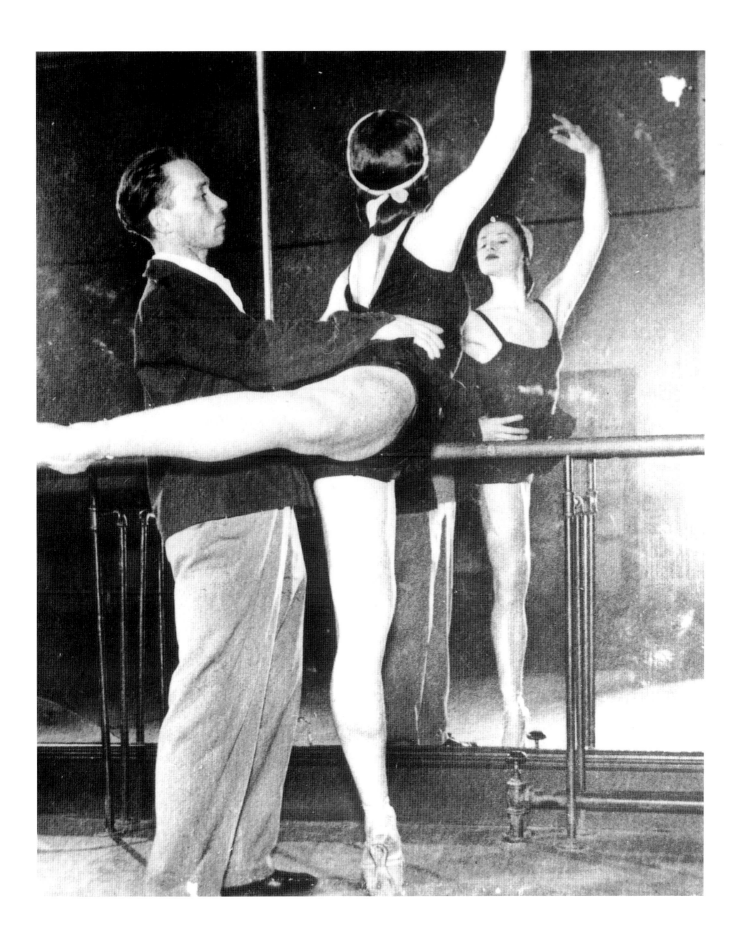

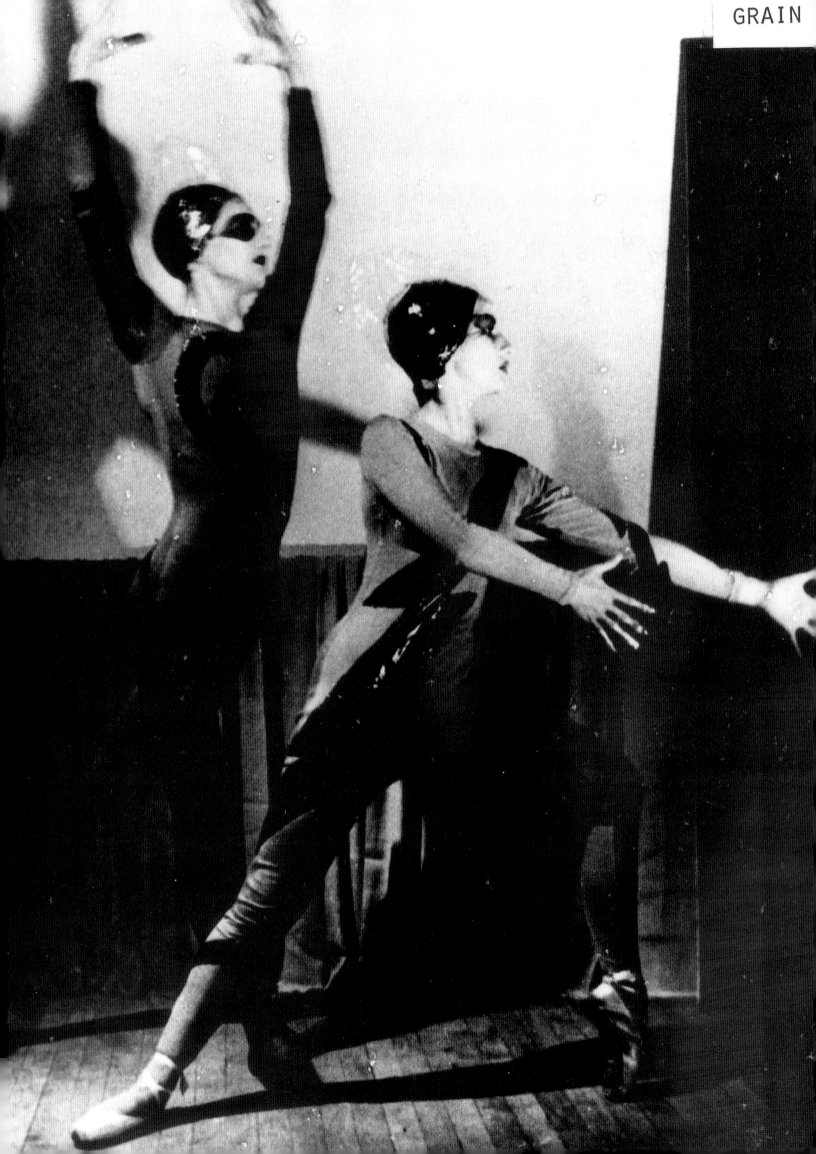

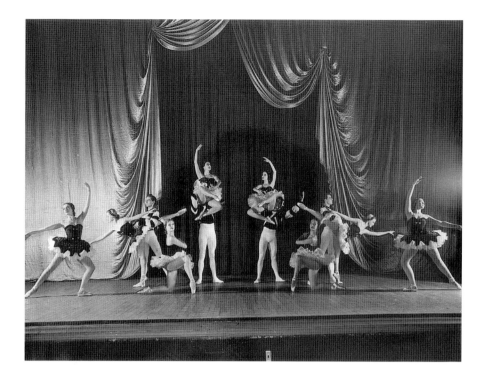

A climactic moment from *Arabesque I,* a classical piece in traditional *grand-divertissement* style, made by Gweneth Lloyd for the Winnipeg Ballet in 1947 as a showpiece for the technical abilities of the company principals. *Left to right:* Lillian Lewis, Jean McKenzie and Arnold Spohr. (Courtesy Royal Winnipeg Ballet)

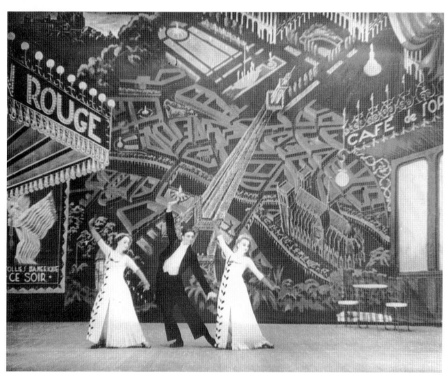

The first three stars of the Winnipeg Ballet (*left to right*), Betty Farrally, Paddy Stone and Jean McKenzie, in *An American in Paris,* a 1943 work by Gweneth Lloyd with decors by John Russell, an early collaborator. The work was a comedy about a homesick American in France just before the Second World War. (Courtesy Royal Winnipeg Ballet)

Facing page: Paddy Stone and Edith Jamieson in a pose from *Kilowatt Magic* (wrongly identified on the photograph as *Grain*), one of the first two works created for the Winnipeg Ballet Club by Gweneth Lloyd in 1939. (Royal Winnipeg Ballet Collection, Manitoba Archives)

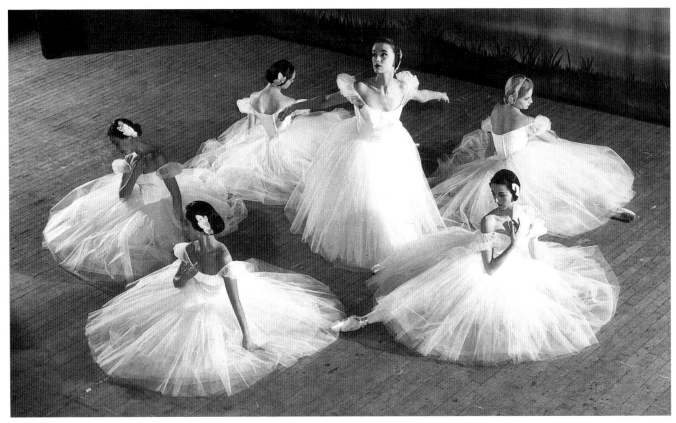

Romance, a 1949 work in traditional Romantic style by Gweneth Lloyd. Olivia Wyatt (*centre*), with (*clockwise, from top right*) Kit Copping, Sheila Mackinnon, Naomi Kimura, Rachel Browne (later to found Winnipeg's Contemporary Dancers) and Beverley Barkley. Like many Lloyd works, this ballet was lost in the 1954 Winnipeg Ballet fire. (Courtesy Royal Winnipeg Ballet)

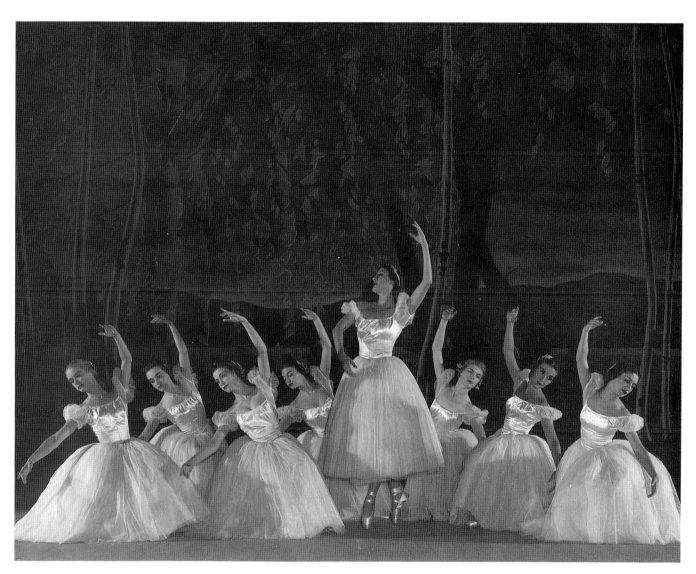

Eva von Gencsy stands at the centre of a group of dancers in *Romance,* a plotless Romantic ballet to music of Glazunov made by Gweneth Lloyd for the Royal Winnipeg Ballet in 1949. (Phillips-Gutkin photograph)

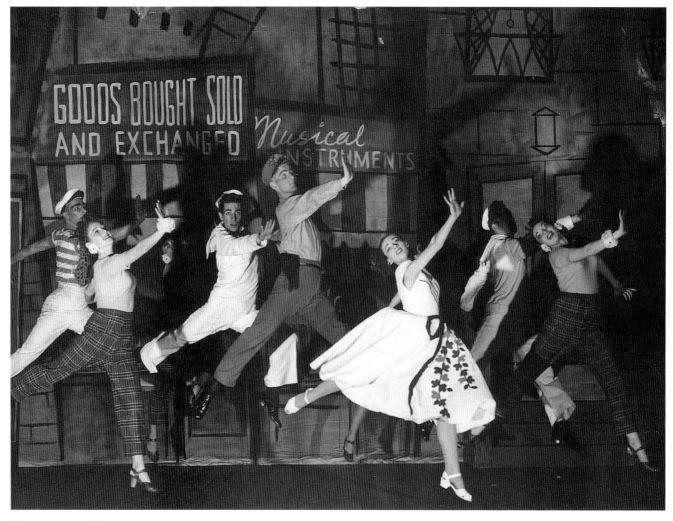

The Winnipeg Ballet in *Chapter 13,* a 1947 work by Gweneth Lloyd based on the popular dime-novel New York thrillers of the day. It was originally danced to a Gershwin score, but Gershwin's representatives forbade the use of the music, so the company commissioned a new score from Canadian composer Robert Fleming—built on an exact replica of the Gershwin rhythmic structure. (Courtesy Gweneth Lloyd)

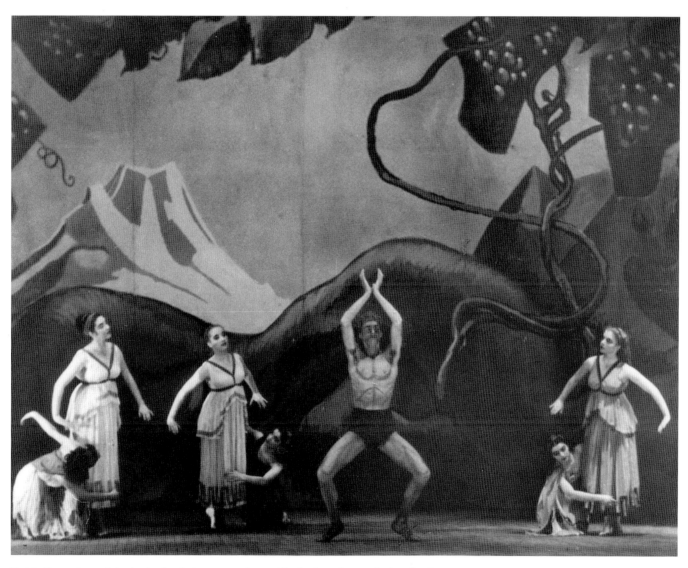

Paddy Stone (*centre*) in the lead role in Gweneth Lloyd's 1945 ballet *Dionysus,* her version of a Bacchanalian orgy. It so offended the wife of the lieutenant-governor of Manitoba that she stormed from the theatre, crying: "I only hope that these girls don't understand what they're doing." Standing, in the role of maidens (*left to right*): Lillian Lewis, Margaret Hample and Dale Clark. (Courtesy Royal Winnipeg Ballet)

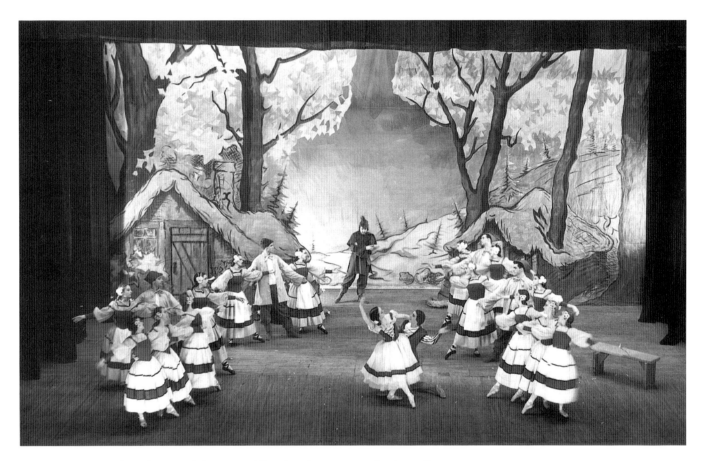

An ensemble view of the first act of the first Canadian production of *Giselle,* mounted by Nesta Toumine's Ottawa Ballet Company in March 1948. Jean Stoneham was Giselle, with Vladimir Dokoudovsky guesting from de Basil's Original Ballet Russe company as Albrecht. The company "binds itself to the classic tradition and thereby fulfils an important mission in the general scheme of Canadian ballet," said Anatole Chujoy of *Dance News.* (Roddy Pasch photograph)

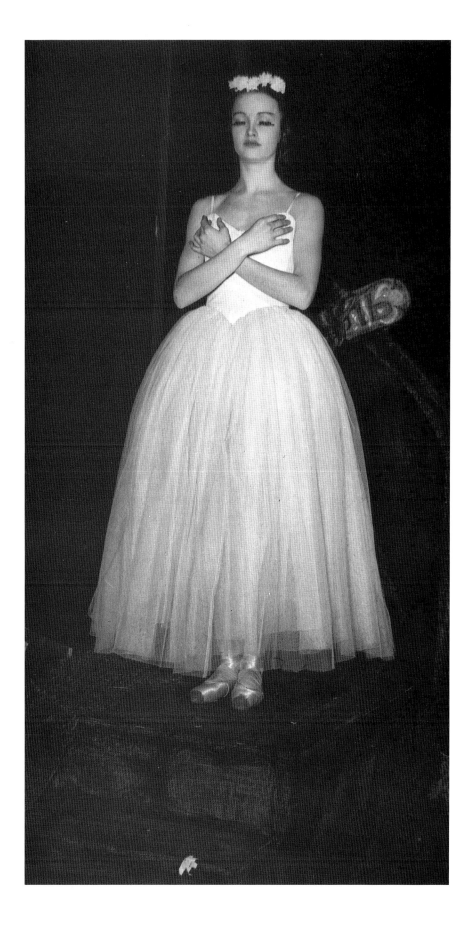

Jean Stoneham in the first made-in-Canada *Giselle,* dancing the lead at the single performance given by the Ottawa Ballet Company in 1948. Here she emerges from the grave in Act II. (Roddy Pasch photograph)

Modern Dance

THE RISE OF MODERN DANCE AND EXPRESSIONISM

Modern dance, as New York critic John Martin said as early as 1933, is not so much a system, more a point of view; there are as many modern dance techniques, it sometimes seems, as there are modern dancers.

One thing the originators of modern dance did have in common was an instinct for revolution—a desire to liberate dance from the formal restraints of ballet technique and allow the unrestrained body the opportunity to make its own metaphor. But the modernists of Europe and the modernists of the United States differed greatly in the manner in which they brought this revolution about, and in Canada these differences of approach have a particular importance.

The revolution brought about by the early American modernist choreographers went beyond the desire to be independent spirits, beyond the down-to-earth wish to celebrate gravity rather than to pretend to attempt to defy it, as ballet did. They were artists who wanted to extend the language of dance to allow them to speak about subjects that were relevant to them in their place at their particular time—to create what Martha Graham called graphs of the heart—and the manner in which they spoke was predominantly life-affirming, their mood brave and adventurous.

The European modernists approached the task of making statements about the world they lived in from a different tack. Their work was more sombre, more inward-looking, more concerned with man's reconciliation to his lot than with any impulse to challenge new frontiers. A familiar manifestation of modernism in Europe's performing arts during the anxious 1920s and 1930s was the expressionist movement. Its extreme passions, emotional freedom and emphasis on immediacy provided a fine outlet for the tumultuous moods of the time. In dance, European expressionism had its roots in the early movement theories of a number of individuals who were not in fact dancers—François Delsarte, Emile Jacques Dalcroze and Rudolf von Laban.

Delsarte, who was born in France in 1811, evolved a quasi-spiritual theory that allowed the body to express ideas, emotions or spiritual states more realistically than had previously been thought possible. Many creative and performing artists—among them the Swedish singer Jenny Lind and the dancer Isadora Duncan—gave his ideas enthusiastic support.

Duncan's own contribution to the development of modern dance was to inspire a new vision of the expressive potential of the human body in motion, and the awe in which she has subsequently been held throws into somewhat ironic light the fate of her contemporary, the Canadian dancer Maud Allan.

Born in Toronto in 1883, Allan trained in San Francisco and Europe, and made her dancing debut in Vienna when she was 20, performing *The Vision of Salome*, to the Richard Strauss score. Like Duncan, she wanted to revive the ancient Greek forms (there was a flowering of interest in matters Greek at the time, as a result of important excavations at Troy and Mycenae). Like Duncan, she danced in loose robes. In her time, which was also Duncan's, she was by far the more popular, yet she was to become little more than a footnote to a period of dance history dominated by her scandalous and glamorously tragic contemporary.

Ruth St. Denis was another American modernist pioneer much influenced by Delsarte. St. Denis and her partner Ted Shawn gave their dancers two things: a broad dance training, and something to kick against when it came their time to rebel. Martha Graham was one of those rebels; so was Doris Humphrey. Between them they shaped the future of modern dance.

Dalcroze was a Geneva-based music teacher born in Vienna in 1865, whose system of eurhythmics was based on the idea of turning sound into movement—"to make," as he said, "feeling for rhythm a physical experience."

But of these three principal theorists, it was Laban, born in Bratislava in 1879, who had, through his pupils, the greatest effect on modern dance. At the root of his theories was the belief that expression in dance came from gesture and rhythm; he was also an early believer in the validity of spontaneous movement as an expressive entity unto itself.

One of the best-regarded of the early choreographer-dancers in Canada in the late 1930s and 1940s, Elizabeth Leese, was Laban-trained. Born in Denmark, she studied ballet in Germany before joining the Swiss-based Trudi Schoop Comic Ballet in 1932. After injury forced her to retire, she studied modern dance at the Jooss-Leeder school and in 1939 settled in Canada.

Leese danced and taught for three years with the Boris Volkoff company in Toronto, and in 1945 opened a school in Montreal. She brought together performing troupes for the ballet festivals of 1951, 1952 and 1953. Her choreography was an early crossover experiment, drawing on the tradition of classical ballet and the vocabulary of modern dance. She is best remembered for an adaptation of Ibsen's *The Lady from the Sea*, first seen at the 1952 ballet festival and later taken into the repertoire of the National Ballet of Canada.

The most influential dancer of this period in Europe was Mary Wigman, born in Hanover in 1886, the originator and greatest exponent of German expressionist dance. (Her work was to influence Canadian dance not only in her own time, but through the example of the European neo-expressionists who rediscovered and amplified her principles in the 1980s.) A pupil of both Dalcroze and Laban, she created a movement form that gave sober expression to large concerns. At the essence of her work was always a vigorous belief in the human instinct for life, but it was infused with the darkly introspective antiwar disillusionment of the Germany of the 1920s. She was one of the first to talk of dance's inherent absoluteness as an expressive art form—sometimes she dispensed with music entirely in order to allow the movement its own integrity—and in that she was a child of her time, the time of the evolution of Dadaism. It was at a Dada performance that a choreographer presented one of the first precursors of abstract, dance-for-dance's-sake movement.

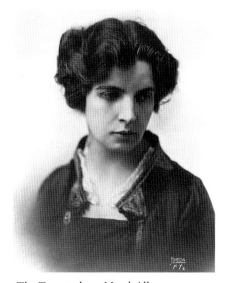

The Toronto-born Maud Allan was interested, like Isadora Duncan, in the revival of Greek dancing. Ruth St. Denis saw them both dance in London in 1906, and recalled in her memoirs that Allan played to packed houses while Duncan drew only sparse audiences. (Dance Collection, The New York Public Library at Lincoln Center, Astor, Lenox and Tilden Foundations)

Across Europe in the aftermath of the First World War, romanticism and traditional concepts of beauty gave way to stark utilitarianism. Walter Gropius re-established the functionalist Bauhaus; Schoenberg, Berg and Webern made 12-tone music a prime force in serious music, and Kurt Jooss presented *The Green Table*, his bitter dance diatribe against war and the politicians who make it.

Canada was well exposed to modern dance in those years. Leading the way across the Atlantic was Mary Wigman and her troupe; most popular, until he became tainted by Hitlerism, was her graduate, Harald Kreutzberg. Also from Europe came the Jooss Ballet, the Trudi Schoop troupe, and La Argentina and her partner Vicente Escudero.

From the United States came Denishawn, with all its Oriental exotica. In Montreal, the Humphrey-Weidman company gave a prewar lecture-demonstration at McGill University, arranged by Thelma Wagner, who taught a Wigman-influenced course in modern dance to McGill physical education students.

Another Montreal-based modernist, Norma Darling, choreographed in the Jooss manner and operated a performing troupe in the 1930s and 1940s as an off-shoot from her school, but the principal performer of modern dance in 1930s Montreal was George Erskine-Jones, a teacher at the Beetles school. Sydney Johnson of the Montreal *Star* recalled: "His work was so 'far out' that audiences were intrigued as well as puzzled."

However, in 1948, the woman who was named in the first Canadian Ballet Festival programme as "Canada's first exponent of the modern dance" was Ruth Sorel.

Sorel, born of Polish parentage in about 1913 in Germany, was Wigman-trained and Dalcroze-inculcated. She danced for a time with the Berlin State Opera and in 1933 took first prize at the Warsaw international dance contest, dancing (like Maud Allan in Vienna 30 years before) a solo as Strauss's Salome. The *New York Times* called her "the greatest theatre dancer in Europe."

Two years after moving to Montreal in 1944, she had a troupe that performed regularly. Her choreography was based in ballet, with a strong Wigman influence and an emphasis on psycho-social commentary. "One must feel a soul within the music and translate it into the dance," she said. "The ballet which does not move [its audience] to joy, regret, rapture or other deep emotion, fails in its object."

The Canadian critics loved her. S. Roy Maley, reviewing her *Epitaph* in the Winnipeg *Tribune*, wrote: "One has never seen on stage an artist convey with more telling dramatic suspense the agony and torture of mental distress when merely standing still with back to audience." *Mea Culpa, Mea Culpa*, about a sinner's return to grace, was favourably compared in *La Presse* to the work of Agnes de Mille.

Observers outside Canada were less impressed. She tried to adapt her style to a Canadian theme, but the result (*La Gaspésienne*, about a country girl's travails in the city) was dismissed as "dramatic chaos" by *DanceMagazine* critic Doris Hering when the company made its only appearance in New York, in 1949. "As for its being an all-Canadian ballet," said Hering, "where, beyond the title, was this realized?"

Like Volkoff, who was finding himself gently but firmly eased out of the ballet picture in Toronto, Ruth Sorel was finding her artistic currency steadily devalued.

Perhaps this was inevitable. Each had imported a dance heritage that was outdated almost before they stepped on Canadian soil. They had been pioneers when those about them knew no better. Now the country that had initially been so receptive was outgrowing them, and the ground they had broken so laboriously was about to be tilled by others.

After 1950 the Sorel company faded from prominence. She continued to dance as a soloist, but in the late 1950s she disengaged herself entirely from Canadian dance and returned to Poland.

LES AUTOMATISTES: Artistic Revolution in Quebec

Mont St.-Hilaire, Quebec. February 1948. A woman in winter clothing is dancing on sloping land in open country.

"All the countryside seemed to whisper," she recalls later. "The brisk air reddened our cheeks. The ground was rough and sturdy under our feet . . . I let the movements come, vigorous in the cold . . . I danced with light feet on the rough slopes of winter, I turned round in the cold wind and ran under the sun . . . I let rhythms flow."

The words accompany a portfolio of 17 photographs that document Françoise Sullivan's Danse dans la neige, *an outdoor solo planned as part of a series of dances for the seasons. Sullivan completed only two of those works—*L'Eté *and* Danse dans la neige, *which she performed at Mont St.-Hilaire near Montreal—but in their experimental use of the art of the unconscious, they were seminal in the development of modern dance in Quebec.*

Mont St.-Hilaire was the home of Paul-Emile Borduas, the leader of the group of revolutionary Quebec artists known as *les automatistes*. That year, 1948, was the year *les automatistes* issued their strident, passionate demand for change in Quebec society, the *refus global*—one of the first visible signs of the growing ferment that was coming to a head beneath the surface of social repression perpetuated by the church-dominated government. Sullivan was one of its signatories, and contributed a long essay, "Dance and Hope," to the manifesto.

Les automatistes were a late Québécois offshoot of the European surrealist movement that had its roots in André Breton's *Surrealist Manifesto* of 1924. Breton, rejecting the nihilism of the Dadaists, had advocated *automatisme*, automatic artistic creation by spontaneous impulse "in the absence of all control exercised by reason and outside all aesthetic and moral preoccupations."

In the Quebec of the 1940s, the province's artists saw surrealism, with its implicit challenge to the social and artistic *status quo*, as a tool to help them break French Canada free of the cultural and economic straitjacket in which it had been kept for so long by church and state.

The surrealist connection in Quebec bridged directly back to France and the

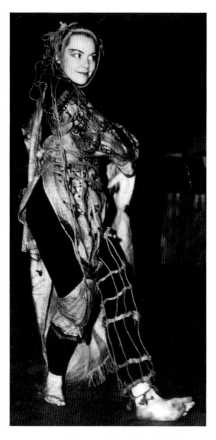

Françoise Sullivan in her dance Black and Tan, *created in 1949 to music of Duke Ellington. It was one of seven short works shown in a programme called "Les deux arts," featuring new dance and theatre. The costume was by fellow* automatiste *Jean-Paul Mousseau, and the text was by Maurice Gauvin. (Courtesy Françoise Sullivan)*

Surrealist Manifesto, via two Montreal painters who had studied in Paris in the 1920s—Alfred Pellan and Borduas. Françoise Sullivan's contact with Borduas began in 1943; she was 17, part of the cluster of student poets, painters, writers and dancers who rallied to his artistic cause. In the fall of 1944, Sullivan went to New York to search out the new dance, and discovered Franciska Boas, daughter of the anthrolopologist Franz Boas, who stimulated an interest in ritual in dance. Ritual and *automatisme* were the principal creative influences on the dances Sullivan made when she returned to Montreal in 1947.

Françoise Sullivan was arguably the first dancer in Quebec to evolve a sustained rationale for modern dance, and her thinking affected many of the leaders of Quebec's independent-dance movement of the 1980s, among them Daniel Soulières, Ginette Laurin, Monique Giard, Paul-André Fortier, Michèle Febvre and Daniel Léveillé, all of whom performed with Sullivan.

Two other individuals who were to play important roles in the growth of modern dance in Quebec were involved on the fringes of the *automatiste* movement—Françoise Riopelle and Jeanne Renaud.

Riopelle's involvement was brief. After studies with Morenoff and Elizabeth Leese, she went to Europe in 1946 in search of broader dance experience, briefly returning in 1948–49 to sign the *refus global* and be part of the fracas.

Renaud, age 18 at the time of the manifesto's publication, collaborated with Sullivan on a dance production in 1948, but left Montreal for New York and Paris.

Almost 20 years after their youthful experiments, she and Sullivan were to collaborate again, with Sullivan by then established as a sculptor, creating mobile decors for works made by Renaud.

Sullivan herself did not return to choreography until 1977—by which time she was regarded as the individual who first defined modern dance in Quebec.

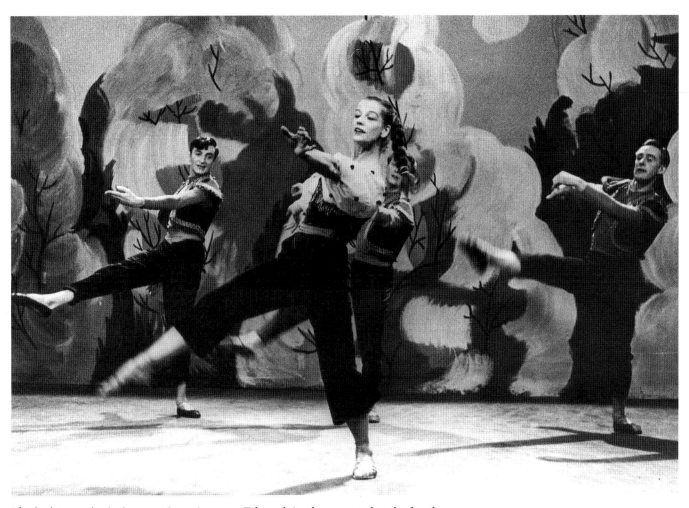

Elizabeth Leese leads dancers Alexander
MacDougall, Jack Ketchum and David
Kerval in her *Mount Royal Fantasy,* a
work to music of the Canadian composer
Edmund Assaly, presented at the fourth
Canadian Ballet Festival in Toronto in
1952. (Courtesy Alexander MacDougall)

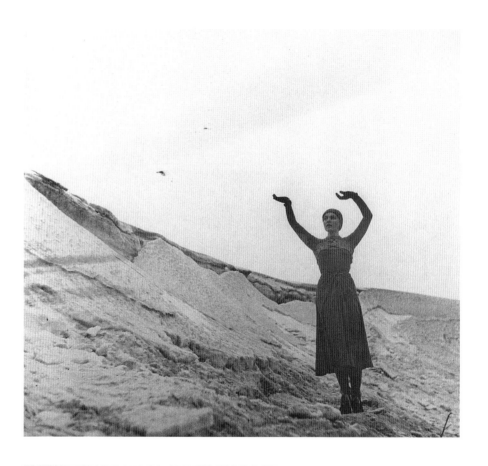

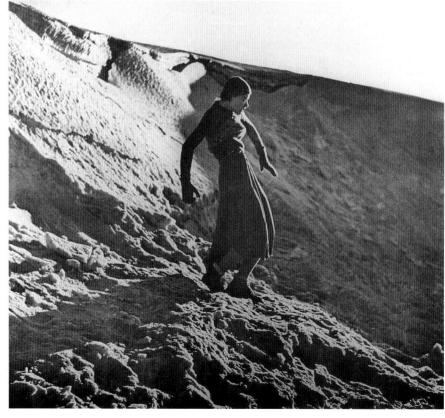

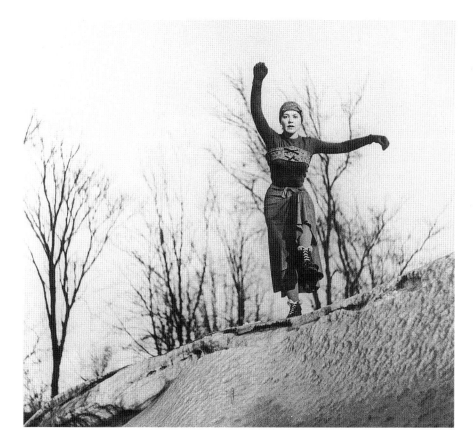

"I perceived the space of day—cut it and shaped it." Françoise Sullivan's *Danse dans la neige,* an early precursor of the outdoor, nontheatrical dance performance that became popular in the 1960s, was performed in February 1948 in a park near Mont St. Hilaire, Quebec, the home of *automatiste* leader Paul-Emile Borduas. *Refus global,* the manifesto of the *automatistes,* contained a lengthy essay by Sullivan, "Dance and Hope." In it, she discussed the importance of ritual dance and the need for spontaneity in dance expression, principles that played a significant part in the creation of *Danse dans la neige.* (Maurice Perron photographs)

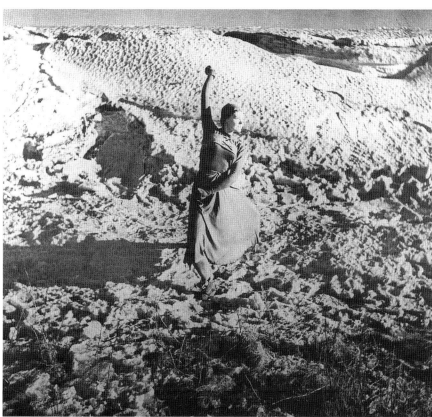

THE
GROWING YEARS:

1950–1970

Ballet

By the time of the second ballet festival, the idea of a national ballet company was heavy in the air.

Logic might have suggested the role go to the Winnipeg company. Of the three founding festival groups it was, by general consensus, the most accomplished company in the country.

However, Gweneth Lloyd and her colleagues were by no means the only contenders. Boris Volkoff had talked of a national company for years. In Vancouver, Mara McBirney of Canadian Ballet Associates (a national organization created after the first festival), was always ready to discuss the idea. In Montreal, some felt the task should fall to Gerald Crevier.

Ultimately, all these hopes and schemes proved academic. Encouraged by the success of the festivals, inspired by the touring Sadler's Wells company, goaded by a desire not to allow the upstart Winnipeggers to hog the glory, a group of Toronto dance enthusiasts decided to make it happen in Toronto. To run the new company, of course, they imported a foreigner. This was, after all, Canada.

———

Certainly, Gweneth Lloyd was available. Despite the success of its first tour of eastern Canada late in 1948, the Winnipeg company had remained in financial disarray. But in its eagerness to maintain an even financial keel, a new board proposed to eliminate touring altogether, and early in 1950, David Yeddeau quit his job as manager in protest. By the following fall, Gweneth Lloyd had gone as well.

According to Gweneth, she left for Toronto for personal reasons. Gweneth volunteered—so her story goes—to raise funds for the education of the widowed Betty Farrally's son by moving to Toronto ("where the action was," as she put it) and opening a branch of their school.

Some Winnipeggers believed she left because of conflicts with the new board. "The truth," according to one board member of the time, "lies somewhere between Lloyd and Farrally resenting the board, and the board finding them impossible to work with."

Gweneth always denied hotly the suggestion that she left Winnipeg because she expected to be given control of the new "national" company in the process of formation in Toronto. Her departure, in October of 1950, was so quiet that for a time the board was unaware she had gone, and she retained the title of director for several years, returning at intervals to mount new ballets. But the connection was broken, an era was over.

———

Boris Volkoff was available too, and more than willing. As early as 1947, he had hired a ballet enthusiast who went by the name of Stewart James (his real name was James Boultbee) to investigate the feasibility of creating a year-round professional company of 18 dancers, with Volkoff as artistic director. The report James produced was positive, and in 1949 he approached a Toronto socialite, Mrs. F. J. (Sydney) Mulqueen, for help in finding financial support. In 1950, however, Volkoff discovered that Sydney Mulqueen and her new-found collaborators, Mrs. R. B. (Pearl) Whitehead and Mrs. J. D. (Aileen) Woods, had sought advice on the creation of a national ballet company from Ninette de Valois during the 1949 Toronto visit by the Sadler's Wells company. The advice from de Valois was succinct: ignore Canadian contenders and bring in from outside the country a director whose artistic ability was beyond question. The group had subsequently asked Stewart James to make inquiries on their behalf.

At a meeting in Toronto, the women outlined their position frankly. According to Janet Baldwin, then Volkoff's wife, the women at first suggested a compromise, involving co-direction of the new company by a triumvirate consisting of Volkoff, Lloyd and the individual produced as a result of James's researches in England.

James obtained a list of potential candidates from the Royal Academy of Dancing in London, and took it to de Valois. She scanned the list and stopped at the name of Celia Franca. "If you can persuade her to go to Canada," she said, "she will do a good job for you. She is probably the finest dramatic dancer the Wells has ever had."

Celia Franca, born Celia Franks in the East End of London, was a direct pipeline to the contemporary English ballet tradition. Trained in music and ballet from the age of four, she was thrust into the Ballet Rambert in 1935 when she was 15, and in 1941 was invited by de Valois to join the Sadler's Wells company. It was at Sadler's Wells that she began to choreograph; her *Khadra* earned 18 curtain-calls at its opening in 1947, and her *Dance of Salome* was the first ballet commissioned for British television.

She became an administrator and ballet mistress in the late 1940s, with the brief-lived Metropolitan Ballet—a company that included 15-year-old Svetlana Beriosova, fresh from her debut with Nesta Toumine's Ottawa Ballet Company. By the time she was approached by Stewart James, the Metropolitan had folded and she had turned freelance. She thought the invitation to Canada "very ambitious . . . there was really nothing; it was a sort of gamble."

But she was intrigued enough to take a look, and in November 1950, a month after Gweneth Lloyd's departure from Winnipeg, Celia Franca arrived in Canada.

When Celia Franca arrived in Montreal for the third ballet festival, she was collected at the airport by Gweneth Lloyd and the Winnipeg Ballet's dancer-choreographer David Adams, who had danced with Franca at the Metropolitan Ballet during his London stay. The women were polite, of course; even friendly. But each was well aware of the other's significance; for Lloyd, it must have felt like inviting the bear in to eat the children. Within a year, Celia would have poached David Adams from the Winnipeg company to be her first male star.

Franca liked some of what she saw, though she was unimpressed by the way things were run. However, she agreed to return to Canada the following February to conduct a nation-wide "feasibility study."

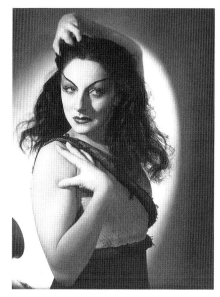

Celia Franca in Frederick Ashton's Dante Sonata, *during her years with the Sadler's Wells Ballet in the early 1940s—"probably the finest dramatic dancer the Wells has ever had," said Ninette de Valois. (Gordon Anthony photograph, courtesy Theatre Museum, London)*

When she returned, there was no money to pay her a salary, so her sponsors arranged for her to be given a job as a filing clerk at the main Eaton's store in Toronto. The job was strictly cover, though Celia took it very seriously, always arriving first and "trying to be a good girl and do whatever was asked of me."

What was being asked of her was nothing less than the creation from scratch of a national ballet company where none had previously existed. She told the *Hamilton Spectator* as much that April. "Canada is a country teeming with talent," she said. "Much of it has gone abroad for recognition. Some of us in England feel we should at least return the compliment, and here we are. I intend to search out as much talent as I can. I want to put on ballets here with Canadians dancing on Canadian stages, with Canadian artists providing the decor and Canadian musicians in the pit."

In Winnipeg, the storm warnings went up. The company was riding a wave of acclaim for its work at the festivals ("Canada's top dance group," said *Saturday Night*) and the town was ready to defend its treasure. "A new company is being formed to tour Canada and no doubt efforts will be made to take away Winnipeg's leading dancers," wrote Frank Morris in the *Winnipeg Free Press* that March. "If such a thing should happen it will be a shame. The need exists for a Canadian ballet company, but meanwhile the Winnipeg Ballet has been such a civic asset that it should not be allowed to die."

The participation of Gweneth Lloyd and Boris Volkoff in the new company was, from the start, unlikely. According to Ruth Carse, a founding member of the company, what the organizers wanted from Volkoff and Lloyd was not participation but personnel—the vital ingredient of any dance company, dancers.

However, one early staffing scheme for the new company had Franca as producer-director and ballet mistress, David Yeddeau as stage director and company manager, James as business manager, and Janet Baldwin, Volkoff's wife, as wardrobe mistress. Baldwin was actually invited to join the staff, even when it was clear that Volkoff was to have no controlling role. She turned the offer down. "I just felt I couldn't hurt Boris any more than he was," she recalled. "I couldn't bear to drive another nail in his coffin."

Despite the sympathy that many individuals felt for Volkoff and his ambitions, there was little feeling that he would have been up to the task of running the company. Even Janet Baldwin, for all her natural loyalty, never believed, in her heart of hearts, that it would have worked. "He was not a businessman. He loved dance, he loved dancers, but I don't think he would have been a good director."

Franca herself believed "he felt very bitter that somebody had come from outside Canada to do a job that he would have liked for himself, but he didn't have the energy or capability . . . I don't want to be rude, but he just wasn't suitable."

However, Volkoff initially agreed to let Franca teach at his studio, apparently in the belief that members of his own group would form the nucleus of the new company. This was not an attractive idea to the other teachers in town, who feared Volkoff dancers would dominate the new ensemble. So the newly created Canadian Dance Teachers' Association (CDTA) deputized Betty Oliphant, recently arrived from England, to tackle Franca on the subject. The meeting was the beginning of a friendship that was to be of long-term significance to Canadian dance.

Franca denied that Volkoff was to get any special privileges or considerations, and promised that when and if a company materialized, she would hold open auditions. Mollified, the CDTA retreated; soon it would take over much of the burden of organization in Franca's early months.

Franca knew, however, that she had to improve the quality of available teaching if she wanted to develop good professional dancers, so she asked Oliphant to help organize a six-week summer course for teachers. It became an annual institution, eventually merging in 1965 with Oliphant's National Ballet School, a year-round full-time academy. Betty Oliphant introduced the methods of the Imperial Society of Teachers of Dancing, which are based on the approaches of Enrico Cecchetti, an Italian teacher who refined the Russian style at the end of the nineteenth century. Today National Ballet School students are regularly entered for Cecchetti examinations, and for more than two decades the school has supplied the National Ballet with some of its brightest stars.

Franca's feasibility study was meant to last until October, but public interest was so great that by June she was pressed into staging a "preview performance" with a scratch company of ten dancers.

They did the second act of *Coppélia*, with Celia as Swanilda, and the peasant pas de deux from *Giselle*, danced by David Adams and his wife Lois Smith.

The couple had met and married during the 1949 summer season of Vancouver's Theatre Under the Stars, and when Adams agreed to join Franca's new group he suggested she might like to hire his wife as well. Franca accepted her on the strength of a photograph. Lois Smith, a former student of (among others) one of the Vancouver babies who went to the Ballet Russe, Rosemary Deveson, was to become the National Ballet of Canada's first prima ballerina and the first genuine national star of Canadian dance.

The scratch show was such a success that within weeks Franca and her little band of dancers were off on their first out-of-town trip—to Montreal, where they did their bit of *Coppélia* at the Châlet de la Montagne and drew one of the theatre's largest attendances on record.

That August, Franca set off on a cross-Canada audition tour, looking for dancers for a permanent company—causing near-panic in Winnipeg. When Stewart James wrote to Betty Farrally to announce the formation of the National Ballet Guild and to ask for the loan of her school's studio for Franca's Winnipeg auditions, the stunned board members resolved to write to Sydney Mulqueen, now secretary of the guild, indicating "in suitable terms that as we are the originators of professional ballet in Canada and have been operating as such for two years, we wish to know what is meant by the *National* Ballet Guild of Canada." Mrs. Mulqueen sent them a gracious letter of flattery and congratulation, and a brief explanation that the purpose of the guild was "to provide a professional field for Canadian dancers."

According to Franca, Gweneth Lloyd and David Yeddeau had both told her "absolutely definitely that the Winnipeg Ballet no longer existed, I think because they wanted to get in on this new thing, whatever it was going to be." However, she said, as soon as the launching of the National Ballet was announced, the Winnipeg company decided to revive itself. Whatever Lloyd and Yeddeau might or might not have told Franca, the Winnipeg company had by that summer weathered the worst of its financial storms. When Franca reached Winnipeg on her audition tour, she came under heavy, accusatory fire from the press. What did she mean by "national" ballet? Was she there to steal away members of the Winnipeg company? Indeed not, she said. "I strongly hope they have the decency not to come (to the auditions). I have no time for dancers who are disloyal to their company." In fact, positions in the new company were offered to Lillian Lewis, Jean McKenzie and Arnold Spohr—three of the company's stars. None accepted.

———

For all her protests, Franca returned from her audition tour with a nucleus of serviceable dancers, several of whom would help shape the future of dancing in Canada.

One was Grant Strate. Franca found him in Edmonton, Alberta. He was 23, and had begun to dance by accident; his father was a vacuum-cleaner salesman and had accepted free classes for Grant and his sister from a tap-dance teacher who had defaulted on payments. During law studies at the University of Alberta, Strate had taken up Wigman-style modern dance, but he had never studied ballet. Betty Oliphant taught Strate his first *plié* less than four months before the company debut. However, Franca liked the short samples of choreography that he showed her, and invited him to join the company. He became its first resident choreographer.

Another was Brian Macdonald, a former radio quiz kid and teenage figure skater. He saw his first ballet performance (Lucia Chase's Ballet Theatre) when he was 16, and soon after began to study dance with Gerald Crevier and Elizabeth Leese. He danced in the National Ballet corps for two years, but in 1953 suffered an accident that abruptly halted his career as a professional dancer and launched him on his long career as an arranger and choreographer.

Recruits were drawn from the breadth of Canada—Earl Kraul, later a principal with the company, was found in London, Ontario; five dancers came from the West Coast; from Halifax came two more future National Ballet principals, Jury Gotshalks and Irene Apiné, who had recently migrated to Canada from Latvia and were beginning to establish the Halifax Ballet; seven dancers came from the Volkoff company; from Montreal's Mary Beetles school came Robert Ito (later to establish a career in Hollywood as a television actor). Including Franca, the company numbered 19 women and 10 men. "And each one of us," according to Lois Smith, "danced completely differently from the others. There weren't two arms that were the same. But Celia got hold of us all and in the beginning just taught us how to dance, really just gave us the spirit."

The company called itself the Canadian National Ballet, which some thought made it sound like a railway. When the disgruntled David Yeddeau, Gweneth Lloyd and Boris Volkoff toyed briefly that first year with the idea of setting up a rival company, they thought they might call it the Canadian *Pacific* Ballet. The name by which the company is known today was not assumed until its second season. The first official performance took place at the Eaton Auditorium on November 12, 1951, exactly 51 weeks from the time Celia Franca first set foot on Canadian soil—dream to reality, in less than a year.

Grant Strate, initially trained in Edmonton by Laine Mets, an Estonian refugee who taught a form of early European modern dance, became one of the founding members of the National Ballet of Canada. Here, he appears in L'Après-midi d'un faune, *staged by Celia Franca for the company's opening season. (John Lindquist photograph)*

The opening programme consisted of *Les Sylphides*, the peasant pas de deux from Giselle, Franca's *Dance of Salome* with Franca as Salome, the Polovtsian Dances from *Prince Igor* and *Etude* by Kay Armstrong of Vancouver. Nathan Cohen, in the Toronto *Star*, never made any secret of how bad he thought it was. "Even making allowances," he wrote 14 years later, "the performances . . . put a severe strain upon even well-wishers' tolerance." Franca's memory of it is clear-eyed. "It was as good as we could do under the circumstances. The decor and lighting were appalling, we didn't have the money for equipment, the orchestra, well, forget it . . . but under the circumstances . . . it went very well."

After that, as far as she was concerned, there was nowhere to go but forward.

RIVALRY: Clashes of Temperament and Personality

In 1951 Lady Tupper leaned on her contacts in Ottawa to win the Winnipeg Ballet a command performance before Princess Elizabeth and the Duke of Edinburgh. Two years later she again used her connections to fix permission from Buckingham Palace for the company to call itself "royal."

It was an astonishing feat. There was at that time no other "royal" company in the Commonwealth (the Sadler's Wells company did not become the Royal Ballet until 1956) and there were only two others in the world (Denmark and Sweden). That single, five-letter word is perhaps Lady Tupper's most significant legacy; it makes the company marketable in places that have never heard of Winnipeg.

Though Gweneth Lloyd had left, her work, supplemented by Arnold Spohr's early forays into choreography, formed the backbone of the company's repertoire until the disastrous fire of 1954. However, the various directors who ran the company in the years immediately following the fire imposed their own interests and creativity on the repertoire, with varying degrees of public acceptance, and it was not until Arnold Spohr took control in 1958 that programming returned to Lloyd's basic principle of beer-and-skittles accessibility.

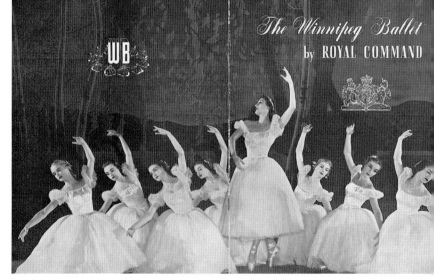

The Winnipeg Ballet gave a Command Performance for Princess Elizabeth and Prince Philip during a royal tour of Canada in October 1951, two years before the company became the first in the Commonwealth to be allowed to call itself "royal." The performance netted the company its largest single-event profit to that date: $2,440. (Programme, courtesy Gweneth Lloyd)

The National Ballet was a very different animal, consciously modelled on Sadler's Wells as a company devoted to the meticulous preservation of the classics of the past and the development of the classics of the future—though Franca always denied the company was a museum, and original Canadian choreography figured prominently on early programs.

Grant Strate, who shared the brunt of the in-house creative burden with David Adams in the company's first decade, was convinced Franca's original plan was to build a Canadian company performing only native choreography, "though she quickly realized this plan was naively out of line with her ambition to create a company of international stature, and it was only a matter of months before she decided to base it on the classics." But what gave the early National Ballet its most distinctive flavour was the work of Franca's choreographer colleague from London, Antony Tudor—the psycho-dramatic *Jardin aux lilas* and *Dark Elegies*, the historical parody *Gala Performance*, and later *Offenbach in the Underworld*.

In terms of performance quality, the two companies ran neck-and-neck throughout the first half of the 1950s. By 1954, according to Guy Glover, the Winnipeg ensemble's style, emphasizing discipline and manners, had produced a closely-knit troupe at the expense of principal dancers. The National Ballet, he said, seldom went beyond cautious, well-schooled efforts relieved at times by "a friendly, though style-less gaiety." But both, he added, were, even in their immature state, "ornaments in our cultural society."

The foreign view was, again, perhaps more objective. When the Royal Winnipeg Ballet played Chicago in 1954, the *Tribune* critic, Claudia Cassidy, wrote: "Royal or no royal, this Winnipeg visitor is no ballet." When the National played Chicago the following February, she wrote: "For the second time in less than a year Canada has sent us a fledgling ballet too soon."

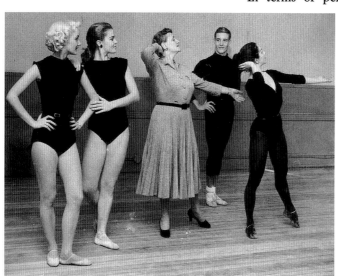

Gweneth Lloyd (centre) *works with students in London, Ontario, in the 1950s.* Left to right: *Dorothy Pearce, Glenna Jones, Bob Christie and Liliane Marleau. (London Free Press Collection of Photographic Negatives, the G. P. Weldon Library, The University of Western Ontario, London, Ontario)*

Years later, Betty Farrally looked back on those notices and chuckled, "Well, at least we were first. I would have *died* if they'd got a good review from her."

As the rivalry between the two companies intensified, the significance of the ballet festivals began to abate. The movement had been outstripped by the growth it had stimulated. The festivals seem to have reached their qualitative peak in 1953. The outstanding entrant that year was the British Columbia company, a collective creation of a group of teachers, and singled out for special praise—"one of the joys of the festival" and "a young Vancouver dancer to be watched"—by *Dance News* commentator P. W. Manchester, was one Lynn Springbett. A photograph shows the girl at a party, her face open and confident, a loose neckerchief at her throat, her hair pulled back. She was 14; this was her first taste of international acclaim. After she joined the Royal Ballet, she changed her last name to Seymour at the suggestion of Ninette de Valois.

Lynn Seymour credits Nicolai Svetlanoff, a Moscow-trained Russian who had directed the Shanghai Ballet and danced with Vera Volkova in the cabarets of Shanghai before reaching Vancouver, for inspiring her to take up dance as a professional career. "When he danced," she told John Gruen for his book, *The Private World of Ballet*, "it was all joy, and I really saw very early that this was the truth of it; if it is not something wonderful, what then is the use of doing it at all?"

By the 1954 festival, held in Toronto, Guy Glover, in his entry on ballet in the *Encyclopedia Canadiana*, states: "Critics were beginning to suggest that the ballet festivals had outlived their usefulness. The period of the dance professional had at last arrived."

Like many dance professionals before them, the principal participants treated each other with disdain. When Celia invited Gweneth to make a ballet for the National, Gweneth said she was too busy. There were clashes of theatre bookings. There were clashes of personality.

When Celia stepped forward at a performance in Toronto in 1954 and asked her audience to help the company out of its "desperate financial situation," Gweneth immediately bought space in the Toronto newspapers to lay out in detail the work opportunities available to dancers outside the National. In fact, both companies were consistently broke. The Royal Winnipeg Ballet lost $13,000 on a U.S. tour in 1954, despite having the British star Alicia Markova as a guest at the performances in Washington, D.C. The National Ballet, touring the U.S. at the same time, found itself stranded in Seattle without cash.

In June that year, the Royal Winnipeg Ballet came close to extinction when a fire destroyed its headquarters, and everything was lost—sets, costumes, original scores, even the notebooks containing Gweneth's choreographies. The company was back on its feet within a year, but a chaotic succession of power plays followed, culminating in the departure of Betty Farrally in 1957. The board said she asked to be released, she said she was fired. Gweneth resigned as "founding director" in protest against the way Betty had been treated, and the breach was not healed until the company's thirty-fifth birthday celebrations in 1974.

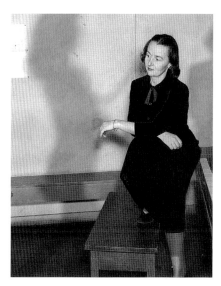

Betty Farrally in a studio portrait in 1950, shortly before she assumed control of the Winnipeg Ballet. From the start, she was the organizational glue that held the company together, training the dancers and teaching the ballets while Gweneth Lloyd created. (Portigal and Wardle photograph)

But if the carefree, pioneering years were coming to an end for the Royal Winnipeg Ballet, for the National Ballet they had barely begun. The company had a sense of community about it, what Grant Strate characterized as "that certain cohesiveness that happens when companies are young. The tours we did were very hard, but there was always an idealism, some of which came from ignorance, but some of it certainly real." David Adams's brother Lawrence, who joined the company in 1955, recalled: "Everyone had the impression it was *their* company. It was like they had an investment. There was no continuity among the dancers in terms of technique and style, but there was an incredible unity. When it happened, it was fantastic, and when it didn't it was terrible. It just depended on the people, the chemistry, the occasion."

Franca was the unquestioned ruler, absolute and autocratic. "She was hell on wheels," according to Strate, "but there was a wonderful side to her as well . . . more so in the early years. Later on, she became embattled." Embattlement was probably inevitable. She was establishing ground rules where none had existed before; Franca had to rule with a rod of iron because without it there would have been chaos. "She was hard-nosed about a lot of things," according to television director Norman Campbell, who met her first in the spring of 1956, "but she had to be. She was holding everything together, and it was tissue paper."

When the National Ballet was first launched, Celia Franca tried, she says, to be kind to Boris Volkoff and to get him involved teaching classes for the boys; but according to Betty Olpihant, the dancers complained that he was always disparaging Franca and saying how much better things would be if he were in charge, and eventually he was quietly dropped.

He tried to revive the Volkoff Canadian Ballet in 1953 as a touring concert group, but it was not a success. He continued to teach and stage performances, but his bitterness finally came to a public head in a 1964 interview with the *Globe and Mail*. "The brand of ballet Miss Franca and her company present," he said, "is of the very tidy, English-governess school of the dance. Miss Franca is bolstered in her position by the hot-air mamas of her women's committee and by some egghead businessmen who know no ballet.

"I am an immigrant too. But Miss Franca has that very English accent and bearing in public; as for me, I am a very forthright person with a thick Russian accent which places me outside the National Ballet pink-tea set.

"Today I am the forgotten man of ballet in Toronto, a city with a short memory and with persons in high places who are bent on keeping me that way for the rest of my useful days."

He produced, in his time, some fine dancers for other companies and other countries, he fought all his life against government indifference to the needs of artists, and he never gave up—as late as 1967, he was trying to launch yet another company, the Yorkville Theatre Ballet. He helped break the ground, and his presence vitalized dance in Canada for two decades. But when the big opportunity finally came, he proved to be the wrong man in the right place.

In October of 1973 he was made a member of the Order of Canada, in recognition of his contribution to the development of ballet in this country. Five months later he was dead.

DESTINY AND LES GRANDS BALLETS CANADIENS

Montreal, February 1952, deep winter. Dancer and choreographer Ludmilla Chiriaeff, 27 years old, nine months pregnant with her third child, has just arrived with her family in Canada. She and her husband, designer Alexis Chiriaeff, have left the undemanding comfort and security of careers in Switzerland to make a new life in a new land.

The Montreal sidewalks are piled with snow. The air is cold. It makes her think of the Russia her parents so often described to her, a Russia she has never seen, the Russia in whose artistic heritage she is so steeped. It makes her feel strangely at home in this strange new land.

They round a corner, and Ludmilla stops, blinks, peers. She thinks she must be dreaming or hallucinating. Above the wall of snow, across the road, she sees her name in large, illuminated letters. The Cinéma de Paris is showing Danse solitaire, *a film in which she stars, made in Europe three years previously.*

"I knew then," she later claimed, "that my destiny was Montreal, Quebec."

———

Ludmilla Chiriaeff was born in Riga, Latvia, in 1924. Her parents had fled St. Petersburg in the Russian Revolution of 1918. The family moved to Berlin when Ludmilla was less than a year old, and soon their home became a gathering-place for the artistic-intellectual émigré elite.

It was a tradition in the household that whenever the de Basil Ballet Russe was in town, young Ludmilla's room was taken over to accommodate the choreographer Michel Fokine—Diaghilev's first great collaborator, by then in his mid-50s and nearing the end of his creative career—and his wife Vera.

One evening, Fokine—"Uncle Mischa"—caught the 14-year-old girl peering through the keyhole of his room as he worked, making up a ballet using figurines and a model set. Ludmilla expected punishment. Instead, he carefully explained what he was doing—and when the girl, emboldened, asked him what it meant to be a dancer, he drew in her commonplace book a design that, for her, always summed up what dance was about.

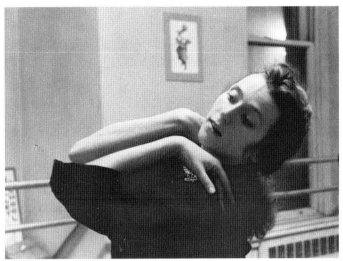

"On one side of the page he drew the head of a man with curly hair, very severe looking, and beneath it wrote *a composer*. Next to him, a man with long hair and a cha-peau—*a poet*. Next to that, a square-shouldered man with a bald head—*an athlete*. Last, a profile of a man with a long nose—*a critic*. From all these came lines that led to a palette, where all the colours were mixed together, and from the palette came one line, to the figure of a dancer. And he said that if one day I would be as musical as the composer, as sensitive as the poet, as supple and strong as the athlete, as self-critical as a critic can be to someone else, and as rich and versatile as the painter's colours on the palette, maybe I would be able to serve dance. That was his answer to my question. I have never lived otherwise."

Ludmilla Chiriaeff, at the first rehearsal of Les Ballets Chiriaeff, in her first studio in Montreal, 1952. (Courtesy Ludmilla Chiriaeff)

———

Ludmilla Chiriaeff gave birth to her second son six days after the family arrived in Montreal. The nurses who assisted at the delivery formed the nucleus of her first dance classes in Montreal—12 pupils, a dollar a lesson—but it wasn't enough to support the family, and soon Ludmilla and Alexis were touring the city's art galleries, trying to place his work.

At one gallery, Ludmilla was approached by a woman who had seen *Danse solitaire*. It was a meeting that was as significant, in its way, as Gweneth Lloyd's encounter on a park bench in Winnipeg over a decade earlier.

The launching of television in French Canada was imminent—CBC television was the first of a number of cultural initiatives that derived directly from the Massey report—and young producers were being encouraged to explore the potential uses of the new medium. The woman was a researcher for CBC in Montreal, and she put Ludmilla in touch with producer Jean Boisvert. Within days, Ludmilla was asked to make a half-hour ballet that the television technicians could use as a training exercise in studio techniques.

She grasped at the chance—but there was one small problem. To make a ballet, she needed dancers. To attract dancers, she needed a studio. To rent a studio, she needed money.

So she pawned her gold baptism cross for $100. It was the beginning of Les Grands Ballets Canadiens.

———

The "quiet revolution" that transformed every aspect of Quebec society in the wake of the Lesage government's accession to power in the provincial elections of 1960 was a period of liberating importance in French Canada. After two centuries of cultural colonialism, it was now possible for the people of French Canada to be *maîtres chez eux*, masters in their own home.

Ludmilla Chiriaeff always saw herself as closely linked with the awakening of Québécois culture. Her own self-imposed task was to help the seed of Quebec self-understanding grow and flourish through the work that she and her dancers did on French television.

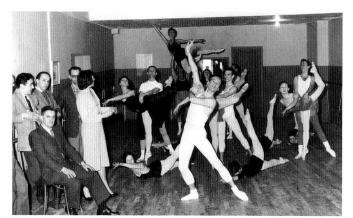

The first company of Les Ballets Chiriaeff, in 1952: Eric Hyrst (foreground, centre) composer Robert Fleming (seated, left) and standing beside him, looking on, Ludmilla Chiriaeff. (Varkony Studio photograph, courtesy Les Grands Ballets Canadiens)

None of it was easy. Recruitment was a problem; she found many of her earliest dancers at classes she taught in Ottawa—they followed her to Montreal, slept on her floors beneath the baby's diapers, and, costumed in her recycled curtains and bedcovers, became the performing core of Les Ballets Chiriaeff. So was attitude—for the first five years of her company's existence she had to serve as president of her own board of directors because no one of any suitable significance wanted to be associated with dance. Parents warned her off—"Go away and save Catholicism"—but sometimes, too, there would be a note of apology: "Forgive us, but please don't make our children look at legs, it is forbidden." The bodies of some of her earliest students, she claims, were bandaged by the nuns. When she tried to enrol her children in a Catholic school near her Montreal home in the early 1950s, they were turned away because their mother was a woman who showed her legs on the stage.

True rapprochement between her company and the church did not occur, in her view, until 1970, when choreographer Fernand Nault prepared a new ballet to Stravinsky's *Symphony of Psalms,* and Chiriaeff obtained permission to perform it at St. Joseph's Oratory in Montreal.

———

Between 1953 and 1956, Les Ballets Chiriaeff appeared more than 300 times on television. It made the dancers famous in the streets, though it certainly didn't make them rich—they received $35 a performance in the company's first year, $55 in the second. Brydon Paige remembers sleeping in as late as possible so he wouldn't have to eat. Studio time and space were at a premium—Chiriaeff would be given a day to prepare an hour of dance, followed by one dress rehearsal, then straight to live broadcast. The floor was cement; sprung floors were not installed until 1956, and then only at the insistence of the visiting George Balanchine, who refused to let his New York City Ballet dancers perform without them.

As French television grew, so did its demand for arts programming that showed the people of Quebec—*maîtres chez eux*—who they were and what they had. Typical of the new nationalism was *L'Heure du concert*, produced by Pierre Mercure, a musician and composer who had been a fringe *automatiste;* of 13,957 contracts issued during its 12-year run, only 534 were for non-Canadians.

As the need for made-in-Quebec arts programming grew, more choreographers began to create groups for the medium. One was Brian Macdonald, who had begun to take classes with Chiriaeff. When the overloaded Chiriaeff was asked to choreograph yet another TV series, she suggested Macdonald as an alternative. Soon, Les Ballets Macdonald were a regular feature of the schedules.

"It was a period of intense learning," Macdonald once recalled. "I look at choreographers today and I think, God, you poor bugger, you'll never get a chance to do what I did, because economically you can't afford to turn six dancers of a ballet company over to a young man—that costs $10,000. Whereas I did all those terrible, terrible TV programmes—which have now been burned, thank God—and learned how to move a group of girls from a square to a circle."

Were they that bad? The critic Nathan Cohen thought so. In an article on television dance in Canada in *DanceMagazine* in 1957, he described the standard of dancing as crude, "a motley of conflicting mannerisms, devoid of individual beauty and ensemble harmony."

Cohen was far more complimentary to the television dance that was being made in those years in Toronto—particularly *Folio*, English Canada's chief arts-performance programme. Unlike its Montreal counterpart, *Folio* routinely imported talent from the U.S. It was also under nothing like the same pressures to define a culture to itself. Ironically, though, one of the earliest Canadian ballets televised in English Canada was Willy Blok Hanson's 1953 version of *Maria Chapdelaine*, based on Louis Hémon's novel of Quebec peasant life. Built in a series of scenes suggestive of the habitant carvings of Quebec, it was the first dance production ever directed by Norman Campbell, later to win Emmy awards for his sensitive handling of televised dance.

———

By early 1955, Ludmilla Chiriaeff had begun to move away from television. Dance had been overexposed and bookings were becoming less frequent.

The first live performance by Les Ballets Chiriaeff took place in March 1955, and the first full-evening performance took place the following September. The programme featured three works by Chiriaeff and one by Eric Hyrst, a former Sadler's Wells and New York City Ballet dancer who had joined the group in 1953 and had become Chiriaeff's assistant and partner.

Like the early Lloyd works in Winnipeg, the ballets made for the Montreal company in its early years were carefully tailored to show its dancers to their best effect. Hyrst's work, though strongly influenced by Russian classicism, was the more "modern" in style; Chiriaeff stayed chiefly with character dance that drew on her own folk sources and understanding, and it was from that well that she drew *Les Noces*, the company's first major success.

Many regard *Les Noces*—which used Stravinsky's score as the basis for a series of traditional Russian peasant wedding rites built around a story of young love—as Chiriaeff's finest choreographic achievement. In the development of French-Canadian television, its unprecedentedly lavish production for *L'Heure du concert* in March 1956 has become a celebrated milestone. And as a direct result of the success of the televised presentation, the company was invited to perform at the Montreal Festival the following September—a crucial breakthrough.

To mark the growth, Chiriaeff changed the company's name, as of that engagement, to Les Grands Ballets Canadiens, though it was not officially incorporated under that title until late 1957. The choice of name drew predictable sniggers. "Since the company consists of just 18 dancers," sniffed Ken Johnstone in *Dance News*, "the 'Grands' probably refers to something else." Ludmilla Chiriaeff

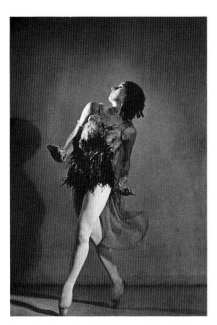

Seda Zaré arrived in Montreal in 1950, at the end of her career as a dancer in Europe, and became established as a teacher and choreographer. Her teaching stressed the creation of line, training dancers to be sculptors of their bodies. Her choreography, using props like roses and scarves, was reminiscent of European modernism from the early part of the century. (S. Enkelmann photograph, courtesy Barbara Scales)

shrugged off the scorn. Her original idea had been to call the company Les Ballets de Montreal, but Gerald Crevier had already claimed that. She tried Les Ballets de Quebec, but someone else had taken that. "So I said, well, I come from Les Grands Ballets Russes, so this will be Les Grands Ballets Canadiens. French-Canadian, that is, not Canadian. Can-a-*dien*."

Chiriaeff always stressed this link with Quebec's growing sense of national identity. Macdonald, a fierce nationalist of the federalist kind, was meanwhile attempting to advance the artistic fortunes of Canada as a whole.

Since breaking into TV choreography in 1953, he had built a busy dance and theatre career, and in 1956 he joined three other Montreal choreographers to create the Montreal Theatre Ballet, where works were to be made entirely by Canadian choreographers, dancers, composers, musicians, costumiers and set designers. Macdonald was artistic director. Elsie Salomons, a teacher and choreographer, was assistant artistic director.

The opening programme offered two works by Macdonald, one by Elizabeth Leese and two by Joey Harris, a Canadian who had been working in New York. All were created to compositions by Canadian musicians; five Canadian artists did the designs. Attendance was small, but Sydney Johnson in the Montreal *Star* thought it "a great achievement that should be saluted with a flourish of trumpets . . . I am not going to pretend that these productions top all previous ballet performances . . . but there never was one that was more worthy of the Montreal theatregoers' support." The following year the Montreal Theatre Ballet gave a season of 11 performances featuring 11 works, seven of them new—three by Macdonald, two by Michel Conte (who had danced with the company the previous year) and one each by Elsie Salomons and Seda Zaré.

An Armenian and former member of the European modernist movement, Zaré had once taught Chiriaeff in Berlin. She arrived in Montreal in 1950, at the age of 40, and by 1953 had opened a school, teaching a ballet-modern crossover technique of her own devising. Both she and Salomons mounted performances by their students in the late 1950s, Salomons concentrating on the new modernism, enlisting the aid of composer Robert Swerdlow for some early mixed-media experiments, and Zaré choreographing in the early European modernist tradition.

The audience turnout for the Montreal Theatre Ballet in 1957 was, again, disappointing, and the company quietly faded from sight.

But Macdonald was at a stage when he needed to create; he needed a company to work on, and the company he had tried to make in Montreal was gone. He expressed his frustrations to Gweneth Lloyd one day early in 1958, over lunch in Toronto. She suggested he try for the job of artistic director of the floundering Royal Winnipeg Ballet. Betty Farrally's successor, the American choreographer Benjamin Harkarvy, had transformed the company's performing look but had just quit the company abruptly.

With characteristic directness, Lloyd left Macdonald at the lunch table and went to telephone Kathleen Richardson in Winnipeg to do what she could on his behalf. She came back with shattering news. "My dear," she said, "they hired Arnold Spohr yesterday."

THREE COMPANIES IN SEARCH OF IDENTITIES

When the Massey commissioners presented their report in 1951, they expressed guarded pleasure at the development of dancing in Canada in the previous decade—"still somewhat self-consciously, with other English-speaking people, we are beginning to discern the fallacy of the ancient maxim, 'No sober man ever dances,' on which our attitude toward the dance has for so long been based"—and they said they had it on good authority that "there is no inherent obstacle to the development in Canada of ballet on a national scale comparable artistically with anything that is being done elsewhere in the world."

But it took another six years, and the fortuitous availability of a $50-million endowment created by death duties on two large estates, for their proposed solution to the various dilemmas of the arts in Canada to be put into effect. Their proposal was state patronage on a grand scale—the creation of the Canada Council, deliberately designed to encourage and affirm Canadian creativity in the face of the increasing cultural colonization of Canada by its older, stronger, more self-confident neighbour to the south.

In dance, the Canada Council's beginnings were modest—$100,000 to the National Ballet, $20,000 to the Royal Winnipeg Ballet, $10,000 to Les Grands Ballets. But the hard facts of making ballet at a professional level were soon apparent, and in its 1960–61 annual report the council admitted that the difficulties in allowing "a satisfactory development of the three companies" were becoming "acutely aggravated." Accordingly, it had decided to "seek expert advice from outside the country."

There was plenty of advice at home. "For the past few seasons," wrote Lauretta Thistle in the *Ottawa Citizen*, the council "has been putting its money on the largest, flashiest horse, while the two smaller ones have proved swiftest in the race." There was also plenty of paranoia. Spohr was always convinced that "the council only wanted one company, and we were supposed to be out." Chiriaeff saw the scheme as one more anti-Quebec plot.

Originally, George Balanchine was invited to make recommendations, but was unable to make the time available; his place was taken by Lincoln Kirstein. Separately, Richard Buckle, ballet critic of the *Sunday Times* in London, spent a month watching the companies at work across Canada. Also consulted were Guy Glover, Agnes de Mille and Fernand Nault, the Canada-born ballet-master of Ballet Theatre in New York.

Although he was not part of the official process, the ballet critic of the London *Daily Telegraph*, A. V. Coton, also checked out the Toronto and Winnipeg scene, and his report touched on many of the core concerns in the arguments over the development of dance in Canada. The biggest surprise, he said, was to find three sizable companies in a country with a population of less than 20 million—"and to find that some Canadians appear to think this is too much ballet for one country." He defended the decision to build the National Ballet on a European foundation with a European repertoire, but he said it was equally important to foster the creation of ballets expressing a contemporary Canadian view of life.

The results of the Kirstein-Buckle survey were never made public (the manager of the National Ballet was offered a peek if he promised not to let Franca look over his shoulder, but he refused), though the tone was said to have been disparaging. Even so, the Canada Council backed off.

"It has been suggested," said the annual report for 1963–64, "that the council should opt for one company, making it (as it were) the chosen instrument of the dance in Canada. It has not, however, thought it proper to apply what might well be considered a restraint of art, and has consequently pursued within the limit of its resources a policy of *laisser danser*. The council believes that if any amalgamation were to take place, thus making possible a greater concentration of available funds, it should come from within the companies themselves."

The shock of the Canada Council decision to ask outsiders to advise it on the future of the country's ballet scene made the three companies acutely aware of just how fragile their foundations were, and identity through choreography was a pressing concern for all three throughout the period of consolidation of the mid-1960s.

———

The first time Arnold Spohr was offered the job of running the Royal Winnipeg Ballet, he turned it down.

It was on the stage of the Playhouse Theatre in Winnipeg, after company class one lunchtime in March 1958. Spohr had just rescued the company from the jaws of crisis—Benjamin Harkarvy, appointed artistic director the previous year, had quit abruptly, with less than a month to go to the end-of-season performances, and Spohr had stepped in to get the shows on. They had been a big success—"The audience got the kind of performance it was accustomed to have a dozen years ago, when the company used to fuse dedication and spirit and dance with the kind of inspiration that had heart as well as excitement," said the *Winnipeg Free Press*—and suddenly the board of directors had spotted Spohr as artistic saviour.

Spohr wasn't so sure. While he had just spent a year in London honing his performing and teaching skills, he had no practical experience at the head of a ballet company. But the board persisted, leaning on his loyalty and sense of duty, and finally he decided to give it a try. What he inherited was a company that had grown away from its hometown public. What he provided was a bridge back to the past—a reaffirmation of the sense of purpose and principle the company had lost in the stormy 1950s with the departure of its pioneer founders. His acceptance of the job marked the start of its rise to international success.

Arnold Spohr is a tall man who has kept not only the elegance of his dancing days (a reviewer in Victoria, B.C., once said he had "legs and profile in the Barrymore tradition") but the innocence and commitment as well. In his 30 years as artistic director of the RWB, he shaped for it a unique artistic persona—young, unassuming, delighting in dancing, always believing that the ultimate object was to give pleasure to an audience. It was a persona that was all Spohr—to do with his uncomplicated belief that the job of the dancer is "to bring good will, beauty and entertainment to all people everywhere."

His programming philosophy was always determined by the basic principles of entertainment on which Lloyd and Farrally had founded the company, but he was

Arnold Spohr, as a principal with the Royal Winnipeg Ballet in the mid-1950s—"legs and profile in the Barrymore tradition," said a reviewer in Victoria, B.C. (Courtesy Royal Winnipeg Ballet)

always careful to provide his dancers with work that let them grow as artists. Convinced that he couldn't provide all that himself, he went on a worldwide search for help—and one of the first contacts he made was Brian Macdonald.

They met in Banff, Alberta, in the summer of 1958. Macdonald, fresh from the cross-Canada touring success of the McGill revue *My Fur Lady*, was teaching at the summer school. It was the beginning of a decade-long relationship with rich professional rewards for both; Macdonald had a company to work on, and Spohr had a choreographer his company could cling to. Growing and learning, Macdonald imposed his developing choreographic signature on the company for more than a decade, giving it character and making for it some of its greatest international successes.

––––––

Macdonald's ticket to international success was a ballet he made in 1962 at the Banff Centre. Its name then was *Pointe counterpointe*; in its cast was Jennifer Penney, a Vancouver-born Lloyd-Farrally student who embarked on a shining 25-year career with the Royal Ballet in London the following year.

Macdonald very soon established a busy career in New York and Europe; in 1963 he renamed his new ballet *Aimez-vous Bach?* and mounted it on a company in Norway.

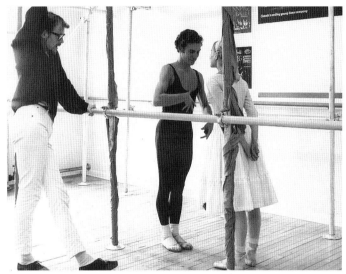

Brian Macdonald (left) supervises rehearsals of his 1966 work, Rose Latulippe, *for the Royal Winnipeg Ballet, with original principal dancers Richard Rutherford and Annette av Paul. (Stan Pommer photograph, courtesy Royal Winnipeg Ballet)*

Its blend of Balanchine-style neoclassicism and cheeky dance-hall fun so impressed Swedish choreographer Birgit Cullberg that she recommended Macdonald as successor to Antony Tudor, who was about to leave his post as head of the Royal Swedish Ballet. Macdonald assumed artistic directorship in Stockholm in 1964—the summer that *Aimez-vous Bach?*, danced by the Swedes, took the gold star at the Paris International Festival of Dance.

The Royal Winnipeg Ballet presented the ballet in the 1963–64 season, and largely on the strength of it Ted Shawn booked the company for an appearance at the Jacob's Pillow festival in Lee, Massachusetts, the following summer. For the RWB, it was the first step on a journey of undreamed-of success around the world. "That's where we became famous," says Spohr.

Macdonald's 1966 ballet on the death of John F. Kennedy, *While the Spider Slept*, was hailed by Ken Winters in the *Winnipeg Free Press* as the triumph of the season. "It may well be," said Winters, "that in this new work . . . the RWB, which already has its crown jewels, its comedies, its melodramas, its trifles, its antiques, its tours de force, its romances and its war-horses, has found at last its soul."

Winters was less enthusiastic about the other new Macdonald offering that year, a new version of the *Rose Latulippe* story, billed as the first full-evening ballet on a Canadian theme. He complained in the Toronto *Telegram* about its "lack of genuine length—a shortcoming which theatrical padding and what might be called choreographic 'prolongueurs' do little to disguise." William Littler, of the Toronto *Star*, thought it a brave undertaking, but added: "The trouble is that Macdonald seems not to have been ready for this kind of challenge. He hasn't enough yet that is new and interesting to say to justify taking three acts to do it."

These were not new criticisms. When the company made a New York appearance in the fall of 1965, Clive Barnes in the *New York Times* had talked of it as "a lively troupe, going nowhere in particular, but going there with a charming zest." The response was similar in London the same year. John Percival, in *Dance and Dancers*, wrote: "It is obvious that the company is to some extent confined by the need to cater for Canadian tastes, which on this showing were not, on the whole, notably sophisticated or subtle."

Canada was not quite in the major leagues yet.

———

Macdonald was not the only choreographer to give the RWB identity in those crucial growing years. George Balanchine gave them his *Pas de dix*; Agnes de Mille agreed to make a new ballet, *The Bitter Weird*, based on music from her Broadway hit, *Brigadoon*.

Even more significant, though, in the RWB overview, was Spohr's gravitation to a woman who was neither dancer nor choreographer, but teacher. Until her death in 1975, Vera Volkova was the leading authority in the West on the style of the Leningrad teacher Agrippina Vaganova—a style that is associated today with the Kirov Ballet and with the Kirov defectors who have transformed dancing in the West, Rudolf Nureyev, Natalia Makarova and Mikhail Baryshnikov.

The unaffected purity, harmoniousness and technical excellence of the Vaganova style was always Spohr's aim for his company, and from the late 1960s he made pilgrimages to see Volkova at work in Copenhagen and was even able to persuade her to visit Canada to teach for several summers.

The Vaganova style, via Volkova, was also the driving inspiration for company principal David Moroni, founding director of the professional division of the company school.

Moroni bases his approach on a combination of the Cecchetti method and the version of the Vaganova style developed by Vera Volkova, but is careful to stress flexibility—training dancers who are as comfortable with *Swan Lake* as they are with Paddy Stone's pop-dance.

By the late 1970s the school was contributing 80 per cent of the company intake, and had produced its first international-quality dancer, Evelyn Hart.

———

Everyone who has been involved in the beginning years of a dance company says the same thing: the pioneering brought out the best in people. United against adversity, they had fun. Later, they always say, the company (it doesn't matter which) became a business, the family feel disappeared and the *organization* took over.

The beginning of that change at the National Ballet of Canada can be pinned precisely: the company's move in the spring of 1964 from the 1,500-seat Royal Alexandra Theatre (intimate, homely) to the 3,200-seat O'Keefe Centre (anything but). Celia Franca had stopped dancing in 1959 (Herbert Whittaker in the *Globe and Mail* called her farewell *Giselle* "a four-handkerchief occasion") and audiences and critics were becoming impatient for growth.

The move to the larger theatre was obviously helpful—the larger stage meant the dancers could give full rein to their technical and communicative strengths, and George Crum, the music director, now had a pit large enough to hold an orchestra of the appropriate size. But it also brought problems: the dancers' work season would be shorter, the repertoire and sets would need a wholesale overhaul (nothing they owned had been designed for use on any stage larger than the Royal Alex); and most important of all, to some—it would change the character and social structure of the company. At the Royal Alex, conditions were so cramped it was impossible not to know everyone; dancers, musicians, stagehands and wardrobe people passed each other ten times an evening. At the O'Keefe, everything became remote. David Adams quit in disgust to go to England. "I felt, why not let a natural growth take place, or keep it the way it is? But to suddenly make it big, how very North America, how very wrong."

The National Ballet moved into the O'Keefe with a bang—John Cranko's *Romeo and Juliet*, a ballet on which the company was to found its mature reputation, and a ballet that reinforced the company's claim to be regarded as Canada's principal producer of the full-length classics.

It was not a claim everyone in the company was happy to make. "We only tried to be like somebody else," said Lawrence Adams later. "The model was over there . . . we used to be told by Celia that we had to educate the audiences. What of course happened was that we educated the audiences very well in one direction . . . it's absolutely ludicrous, because it's nothing but another piece of bastardized imported culture, that's the joke of it. And of course, you can't go back. But at the beginning we could have gone anywhere."

———

The National Ballet School in Toronto became fully autonomous in 1963, and was to become, in the words of Lincoln Kirstein, "the equal in essence of the Kirov School in Leningrad and the Royal Ballet School in England." Its founder, Betty Oliphant, became so highly regarded that she was invited to restructure the schools of both the Royal Swedish and the Royal Danish ballets. Mikhail Baryshnikov donated his first earnings in the West—$2,000 for an appearance with the National Ballet of Canada—to the school.

The school's first graduates entered the National Ballet company in 1965. Among them were Veronica Tennant, taken in at principal level to dance Juliet, and a company leader until her retirement in 1989; and Martine van Hamel, gold medal winner at the Varna international contest in 1966 and later a principal with American Ballet Theatre.

This was the beginning of the National Ballet "look"—an unmannered style, deliberately pure, with a somewhat remote correctness. "We were a great rehearsal company," Tennant recalls, "but not a great performing company. We spent a lot of time in rehearsal—we were very finely honed and groomed—then we'd get out on stage and you'd just sense a stage fright."

Since that first graduating class, the school has provided a regular flow of dancers for the National Ballet (among them two generations of principals—Karen Kain and her longtime partner Frank Augustyn, Vanessa Harwood, Nadia Potts, Kimberly Glasco, Kim Lightheart, Sabina Allemann, Jeremy Ransom and Rex Harrington), but it also takes pride in turning out graduates who are consistently able to find work with international ballet companies carrying broad-based repertoires.

For the 1964–65 season Erik Bruhn was invited to stage *La Sylphide,* the Taglioni ballet of the 1830s that had initiated the Romantic movement in dance. The invitation was a calculated gamble. The Royal Danish Ballet's version, created by August Bournonville out of what he remembered of the original, had provided Bruhn with a particularly successful role as James, the farmer who loses his bride-to-be for the sake of a sylph that only he can see. Bruhn had never produced a major classic, and confessed later that the prospect "scared the wits out of me," but the production turned out to be what *Dance News* termed "an unqualified triumph." Bruhn danced the role of James at opening night, opposite Lynn Seymour as the sylphide. Franca (Bruhn's former colleague from the Metropolitan Ballet in London in the late 1940s) came back to the stage to perform the mime role of Madge, the evil witch who brings about all the unhappiness.

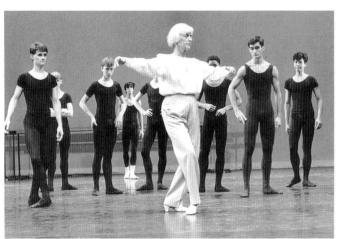

Betty Oliphant, artistic director and ballet principal of the National Ballet School, teaches the senior boys' class in 1988. One of very few Westerners to have been invited to teach the graduating class of the Bolshoi school in Moscow, she retired in 1989. (Robert C. Ragsdale, frps, photograph)

At the second performance, Bruhn injured his knee, and his friend Rudolf Nureyev, who had flown in for the premiere, stepped in and danced the part at two days' notice. The press, and audience, went wild.

The production was the start of one of the most fruitful artistic relationships in Canadian ballet.

In Montreal, Les Grands Ballets, charged with the task of presenting the first dance performances at Montreal's prestigious Place des Arts, was faced with a challenge similar to Franca's when she made the move to the O'Keefe: larger sets, more dancers, bigger productions.

Chiriaeff's response was essentially the same—she went abroad for help, inviting Anton Dolin, the former Diaghilev dancer, to stage his remounting of Pugni's *Le Pas de quatre,* the famous 1845 showpiece for Europe's four great rival ballerinas of the period.

And, exactly as in Toronto, the change to a larger theatre changed the company's character. It was a dismaying experience for Chiriaeff. "Suddenly, that precious jewel wasn't there any more. We brought people in from New York and it was just a job to them . . . we were surpassed by the Place des Arts . . . it was not us; it was someone who had put on too big a suit. I knew that, but I had to do it to my child, otherwise we would have atrophied."

Herbert Whittaker, in the *Globe and Mail,* said the condition of Les Grands Ballets epitomized the basic dilemma of the Canadian ballet ensemble. "While it may not be essentially French or very Grand it is undeniably Canadian—an aggregation made up of borrowed ballets and borrowed styles, but with problems all its own."

What turned it all around was the arrival, in 1965, of a choreographer who was to mould the company's image and influence—Fernand Nault.

Nault grew up in poverty in religious, Francophone East Montreal. His family intended him for the priesthood; young Fernand saw his sister dancing the Charleston and decided he would rather be a dancer. When he finally announced to his family that he wanted to be another Fred Astaire, he once recalled, "many

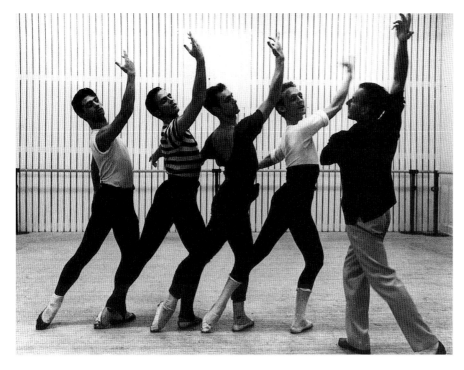

*Anton Dolin became artistic advisor to Les Grands Ballets Canadiens in 1963, the year the company inaugurated the dance programme at Montreal's new Place des Arts. He subsequently mounted a number of ballets on the company. He is shown here (*right*) in the mid-1960s, rehearsing (*left to right*) Armando Jorge, Vincent Warren, Lawrence Haider and Peter Saul. (*Courtesy Les Grands Ballets Canadiens*)*

novenas were said, many candles burned on my account." Anton Dolin auditioned him for Ballet Theatre in 1944, and he stayed with the New York company for 20 years, many of them as ballet master.

Chiriaeff invited him to stage a *Nutcracker* for Les Grands for the 1964 Christmas season, and he was impressed by what he found. If there had been a company like that in Montreal when he was young, he said, he would never have had to leave.

Nault joined the company in the summer of 1965, as assistant artistic director, free to create whatever he liked. "Grands Ballets Truly Grands," said the headline on Sydney Johnson's Montreal *Star* review of Nault's *Nutcracker*.

Well, at last.

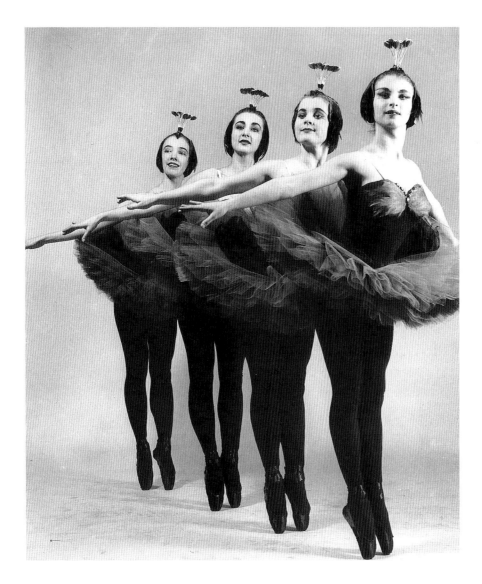

Swan Lake, Act II, entered the repertoire of the National Ballet of Canada in the company's third season, 1953–54. A full version of the ballet was acquired the following year. *Left to right:* Marilyn Rollo, Sylvia Mason, Joan Stuart and Betty Pope. (Ken Bell photograph)

Facing page: Celia Franca with Earl Kraul in the National Ballet of Canada's early version of *Coppélia, Act II.* (Courtesy National Ballet of Canada)

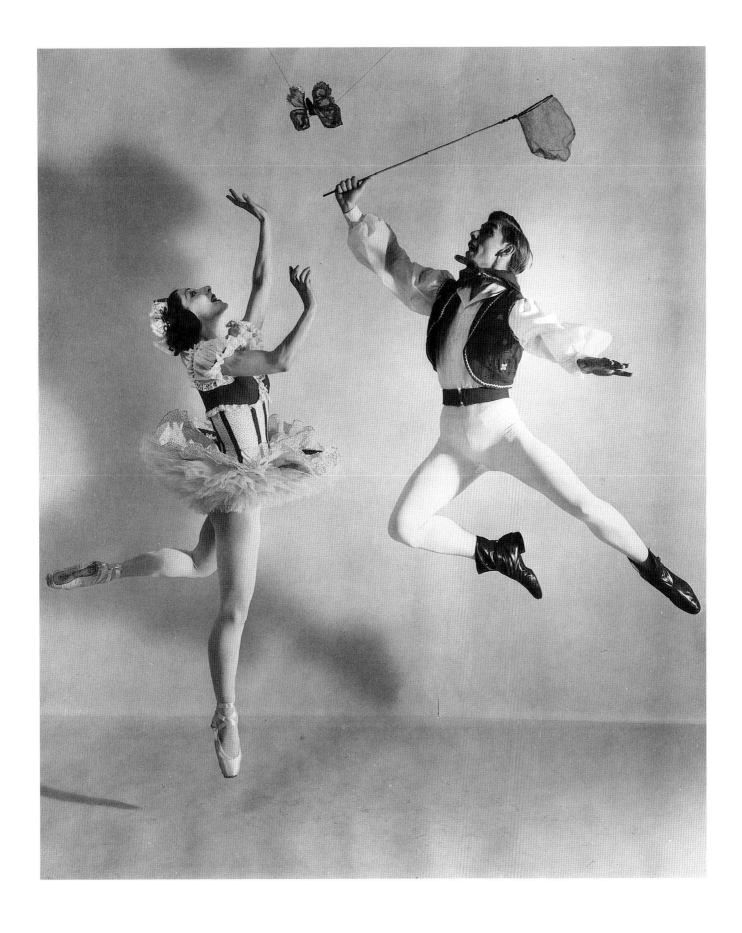

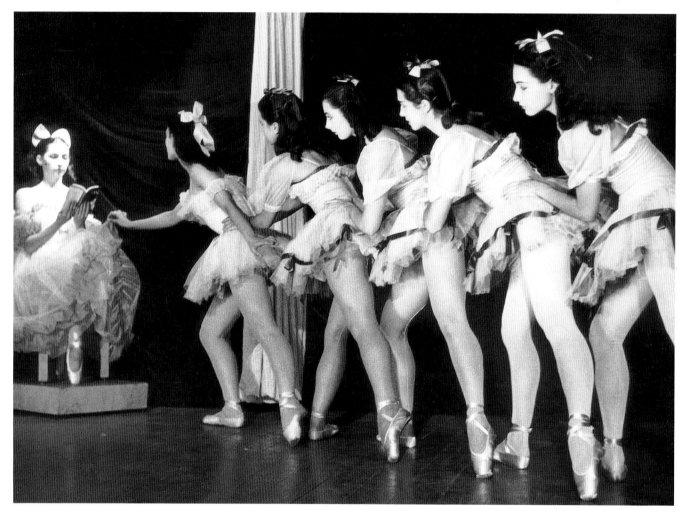

Celia Franca as Swanilda leads (*left to right*) Joyce Hill, Sandra Francis, Colleen Kenney and Myrna Aaron towards Coppélia, the girl with the enamel eyes, in a National Ballet of Canada promenade concert presentation in the 1952–53 season. (John-Grange Photography, courtesy National Ballet of Canada)

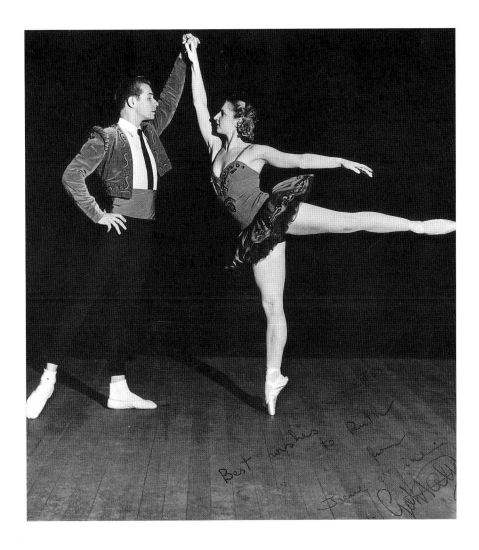

Jury Gotshalks and Irene Apiné immigrated to Canada in 1947 and settled in Halifax, where they launched the Halifax Ballet. However, in 1951 they joined the National Ballet of Canada, and became two of the company's earliest principal dancers. (Courtesy Ruth Carse)

Overleaf: Celia Franca's version of *L'Après-midi d'un faune* was one of 10 works presented in the first season of the National Ballet of Canada, 1951–52. At the centre of this grouping are Lilian Jarvis and Grant Strate (the Faun). (Ken Bell photograph)

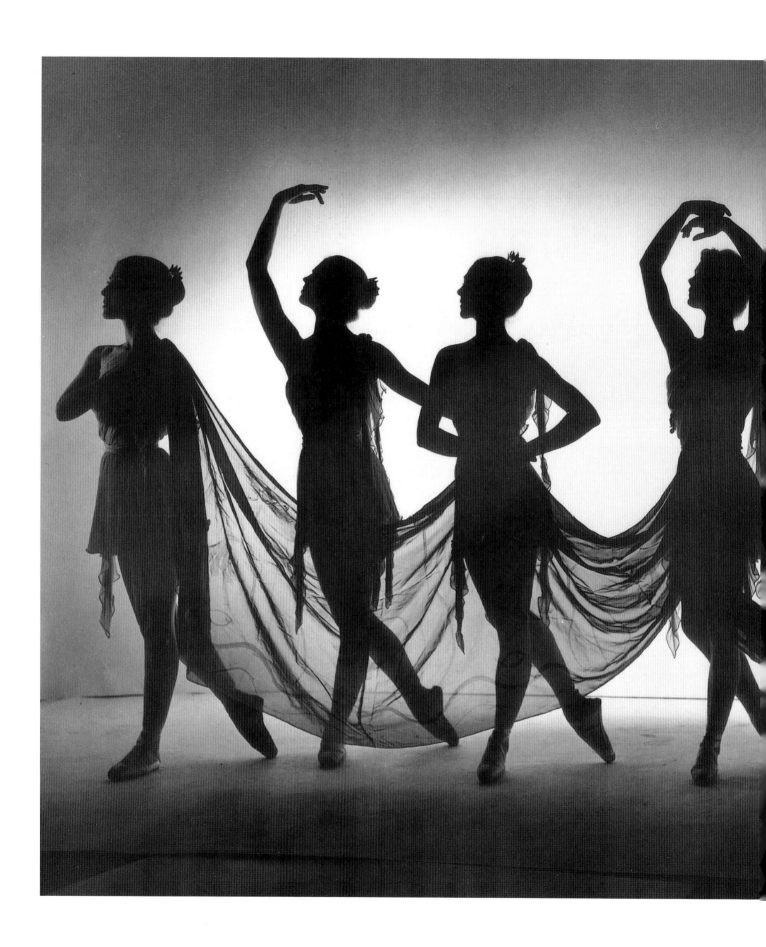

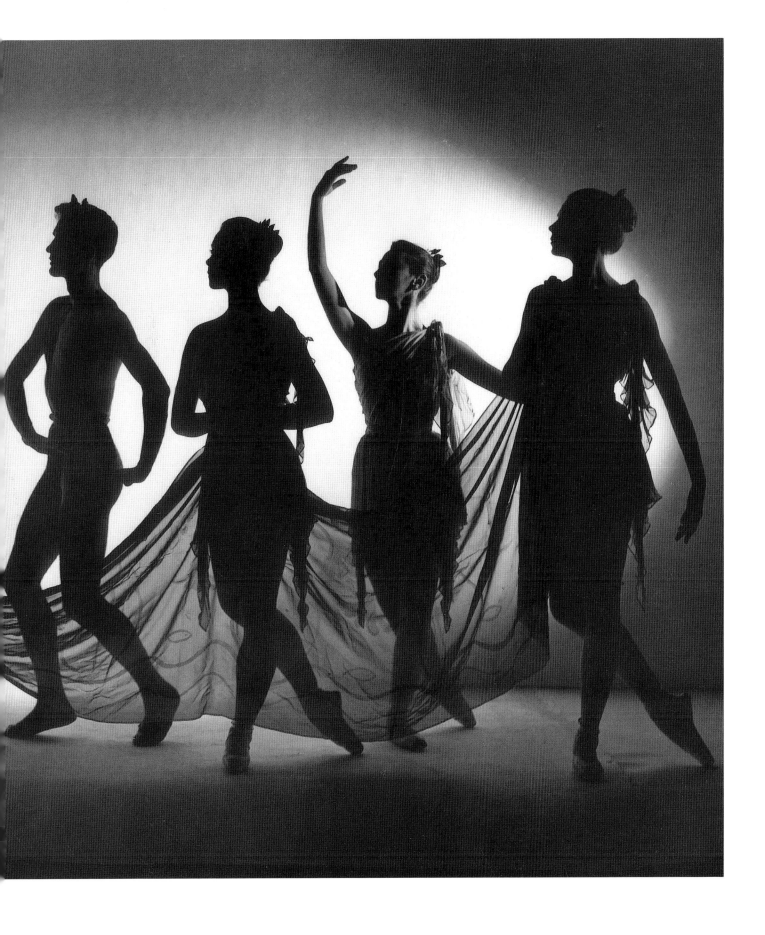

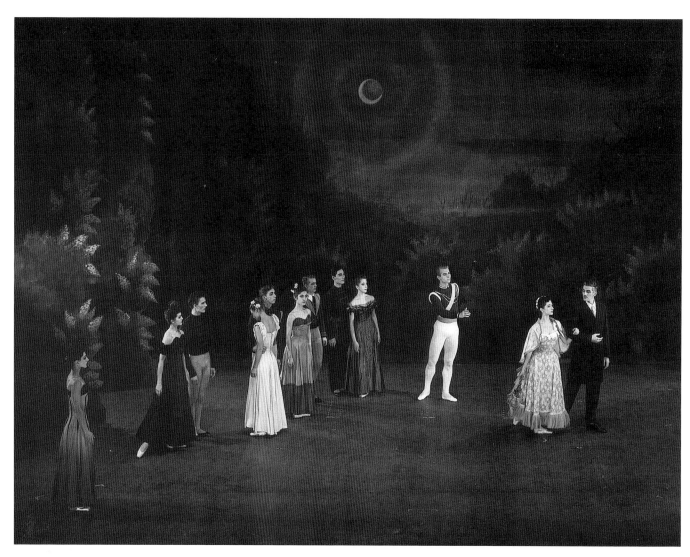

Antony Tudor's *Jardin aux lilas (Lilac Garden)* was acquired by the National Ballet of Canada in its second season. *Left to right:* Celia Franca, Colleen Kenney, Grant Strate, Lilian Jarvis, Earl Kraul, Judie Colpman, Glenn Gibson, Robert Ito, Diane Childerhose, David Adams, Lois Smith and James Ronaldson. (Ken Bell photograph)

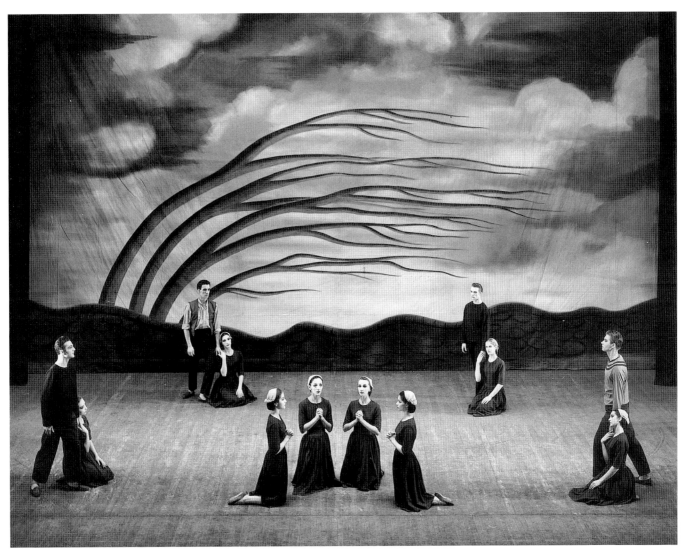

Dark Elegies, Antony Tudor's sorrowing and moving response to Mahler's *Kindertotenlieder,* was acquired by the National Ballet of Canada in 1955. Celia Franca is kneeling (*second from left*); David Adams is standing (*right*). (Ken Bell photograph)

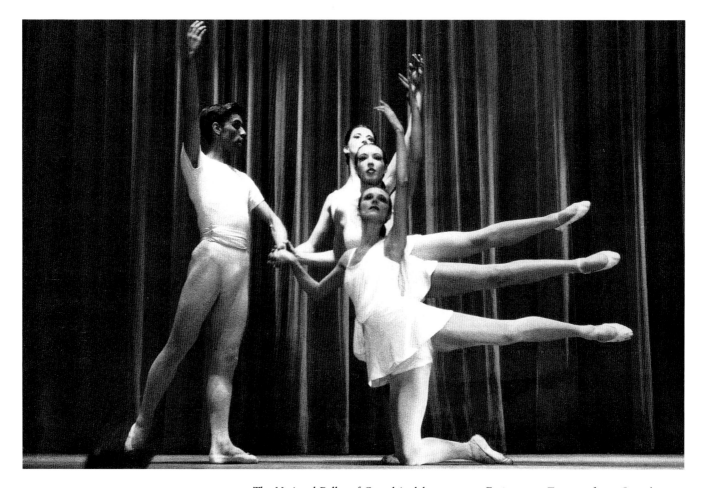

The National Ballet of Canada's debut performance on 12 November 1951, in Toronto, included *Etude,* a work by Vancouver's Kay Armstrong. The original cast (*left to right*): Earl Kraul, Natalia Butko, Maria Dynowska and Katharine Stewart. (Gene Draper photograph, courtesy National Ballet of Canada)

Facing page: Extracts from *Coppélia* were danced by the National Ballet of Canada from its earliest days, but a full version of the ballet was not presented until 1958. Shown here in 1961 is the husband and wife team of Lois Smith and David Adams in the pas de deux from the third act. (Ken Bell photograph)

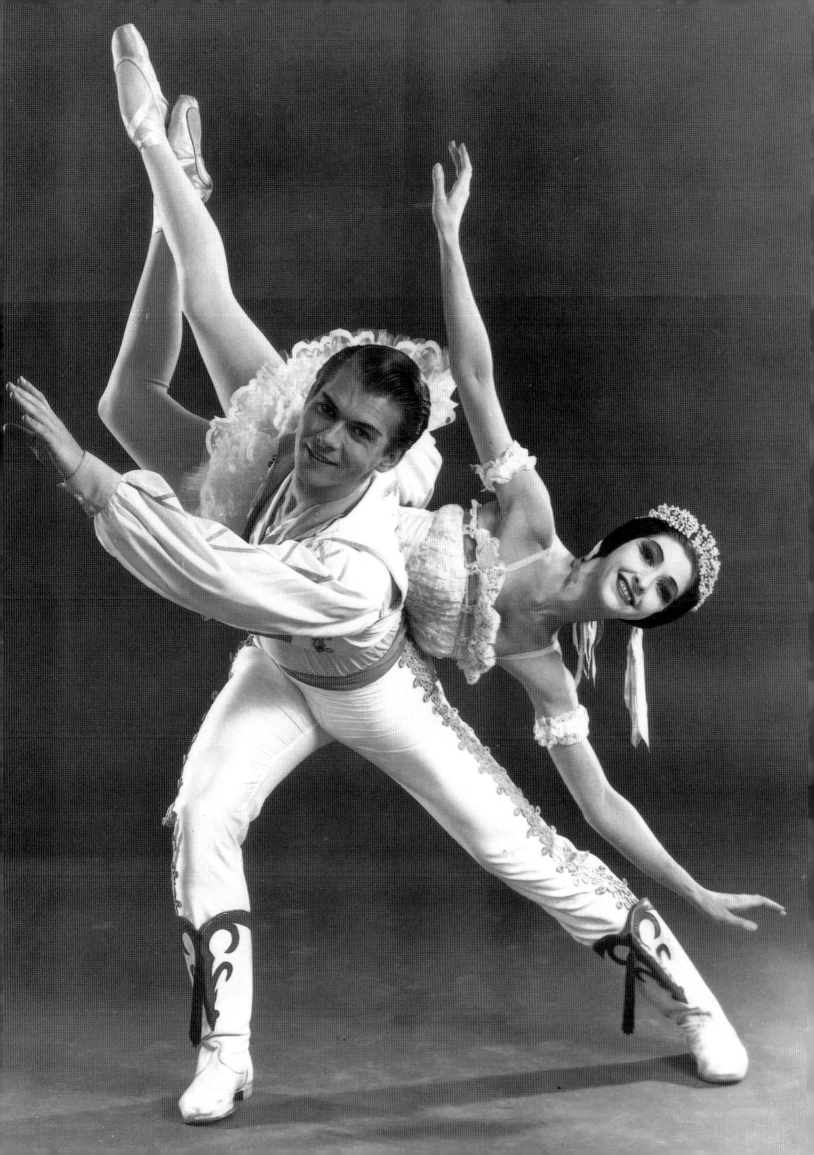

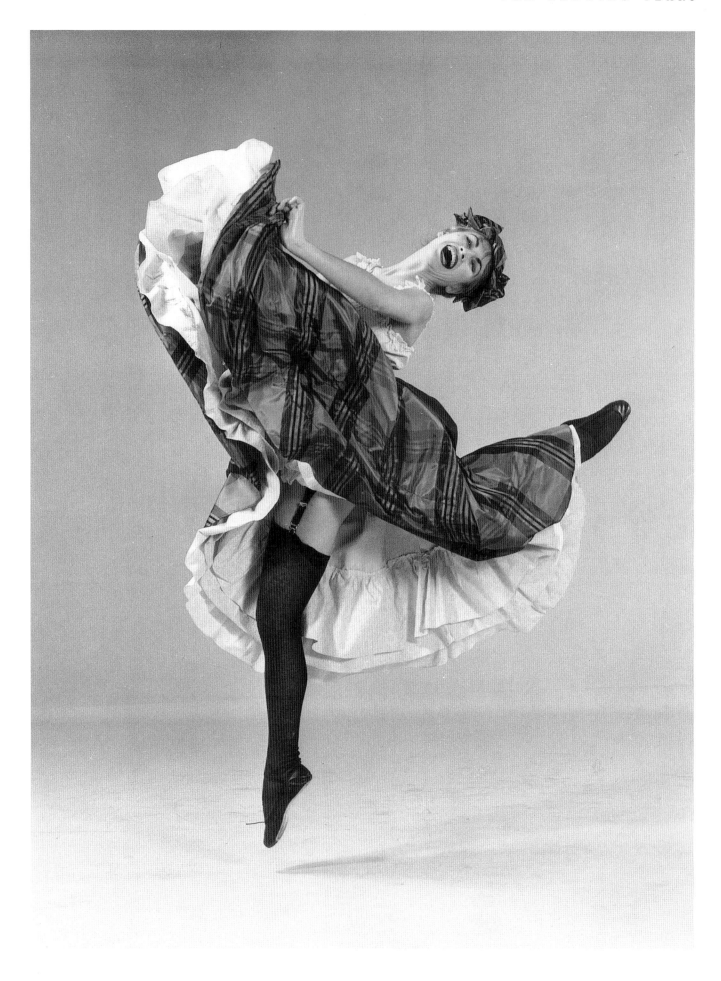

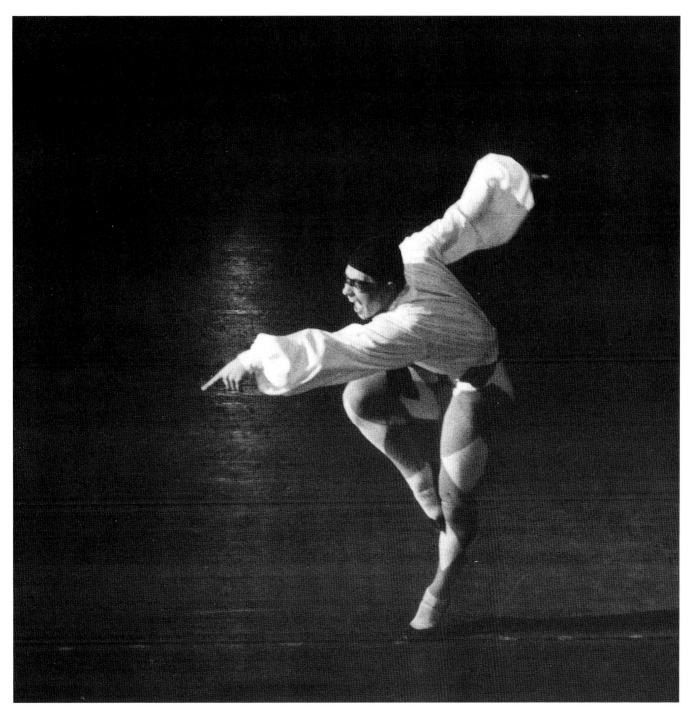

Facing page: Jacqueline Ivings kicks up her heels as one of the cancan girls in Antony Tudor's *Offenbach in the Underworld,* an 1870s frolic in a fashionable Paris café, made for the National Ballet of Canada in 1955. (Ken Bell photograph)

Le Carnaval, regarded as one of the masterworks of Michel Fokine, entered the repertoire of the National Ballet of Canada in 1957. David Adams appeared as Harlequin, a role danced by Nijinsky at the work's premiere in Paris in 1910. (Ken Bell photograph)

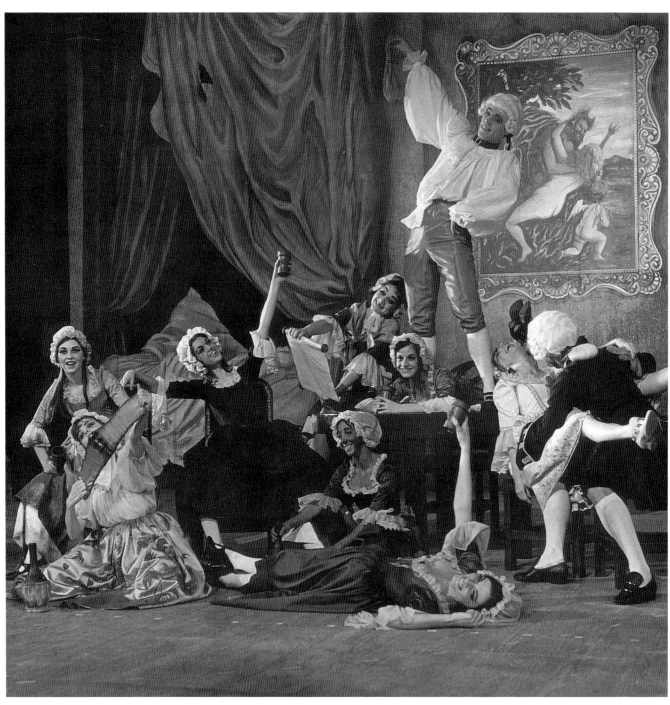

The Rake's Progress, made by Ninette de Valois in London in 1935, entered the repertoire of the National Ballet of Canada 30 years later. "Thank God de Valois never came," said Lawrence Adams, shown standing on the table. "It was like doing a 1930s movie. We just changed things all the time." (Ken Bell photograph)

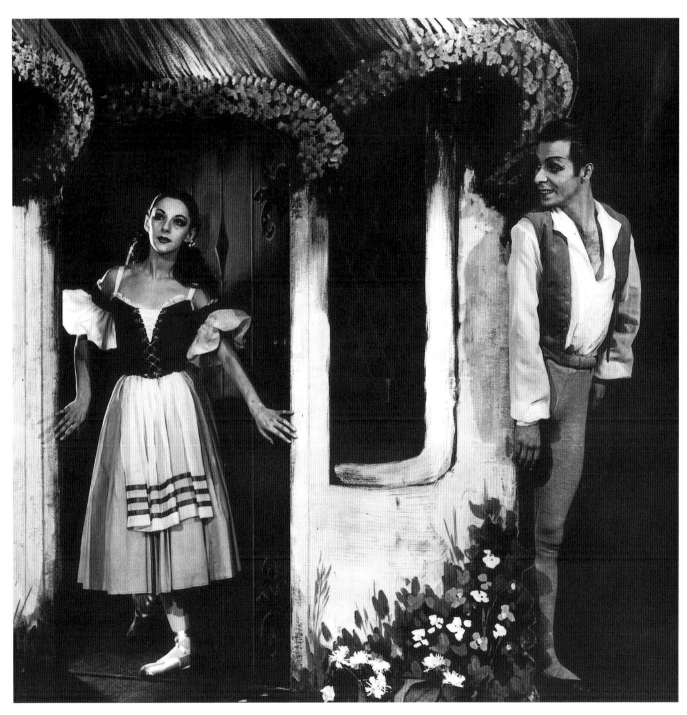

Celia Franca with Jury Gotshalks in the
National Ballet of Canada's early version
of *Coppélia* in 1953. (Ken Bell
photograph)

Veronica Tennant made her debut as a principal dancer with the National Ballet of Canada in the role of Juliet after graduating from the National Ballet School in 1965. She is shown in *Cinderella* the same year. (Ken Bell photogaph)

Facing page: Lynn Seymour was one of a number of guest performers invited to dance with the National Ballet of Canada in the 1960s. She performed the central role of Effie, the heroine of *La Sylphide,* with Erik Bruhn at the premiere of his 1964 production. (Reg Innell photograph)

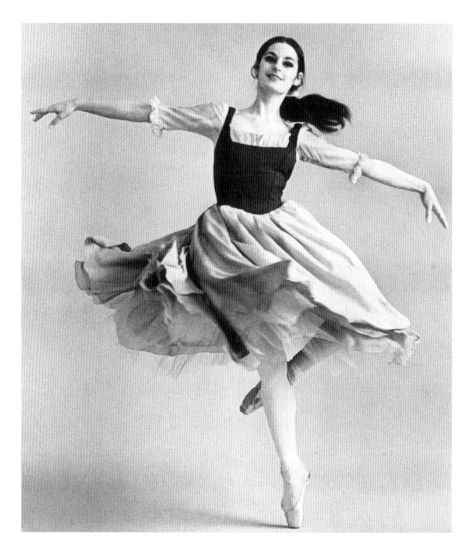

The story of Barbara Allen has been told twice at the National Ballet of Canada. Joey Harris's *Dark of the Moon* was shown in 1953. Seven years later David Adams made *Barbara Allen,* to the same Louis Applebaum score. Adams, who danced the Witch Boy in both versions, appears here in his own, with Pearl Sollère and Irene Apiné. (Ken Bell photograph)

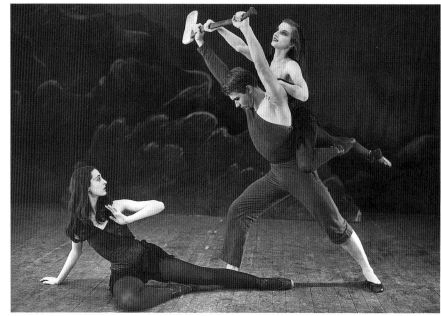

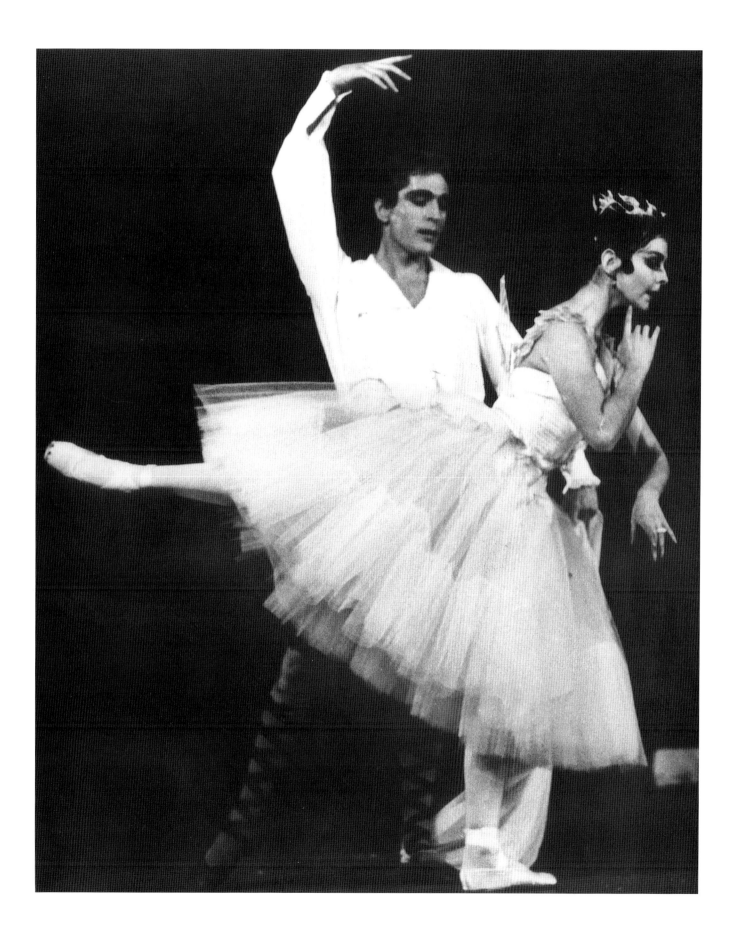

La Sylphide, the ballet that launched
Romanticism in dance in 1832, was
mounted for the National Ballet of
Canada in 1964 by Erik Bruhn. Celia
Franca, who had retired from dancing in
1959, returned to the stage to perform the
role of Madge, the witch. (Ken Bell
photograph)

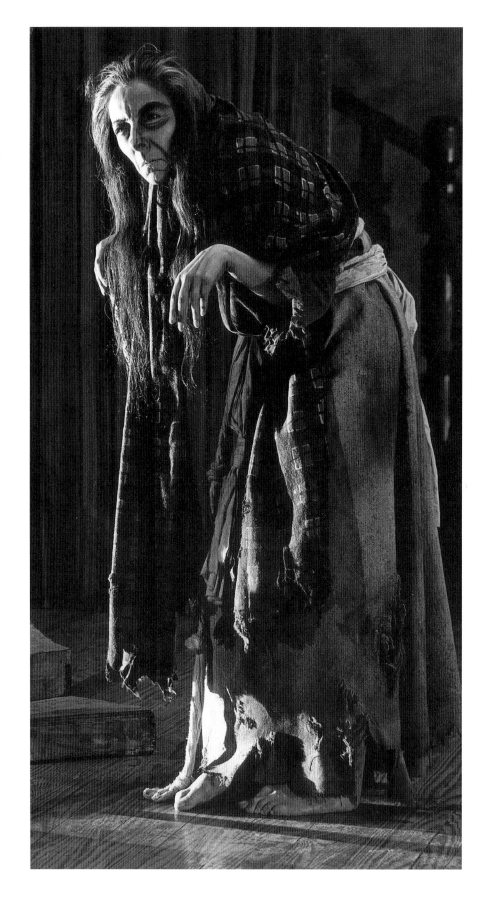

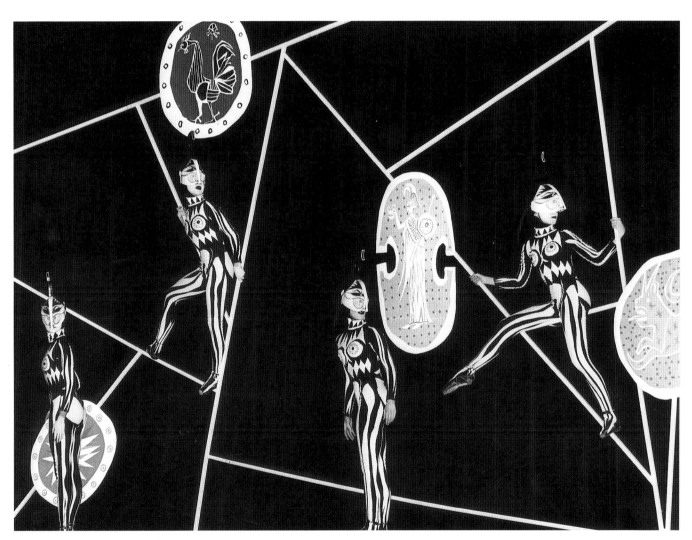

Grant Strate made over a dozen ballets for the National Ballet of Canada. *The House of Atreus,* using music by Canadian composer Harry Somers and design by Canadian artist Harold Town, was introduced in 1964. Part of the set (shown here) was a web of shields and steel struts on which the dancers balanced. (Ken Bell photograph)

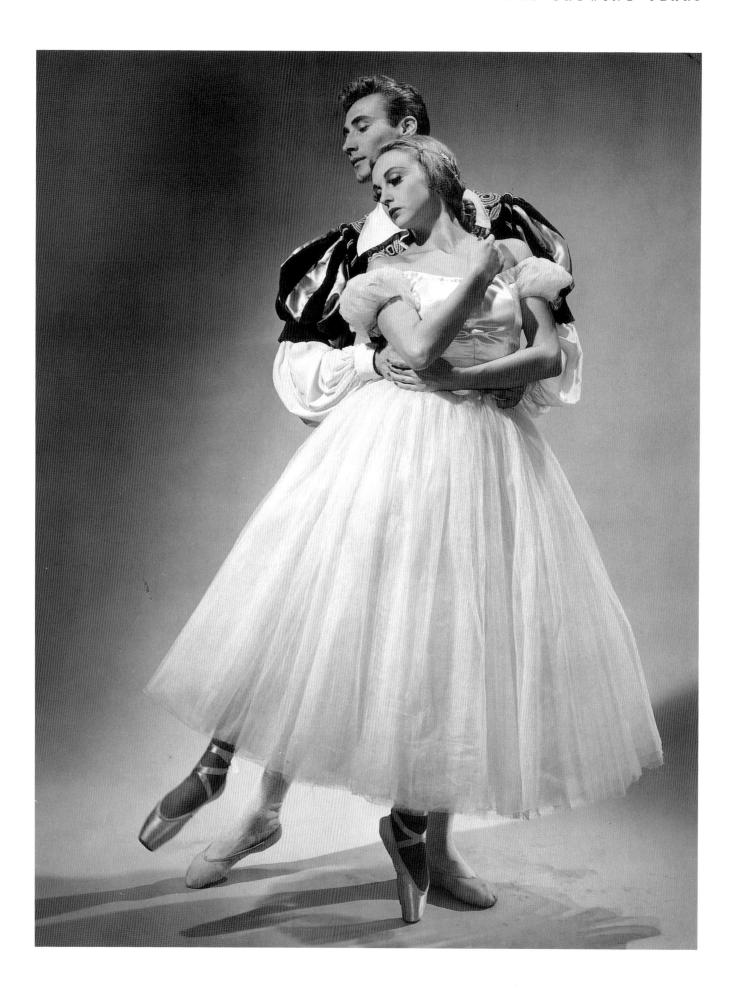

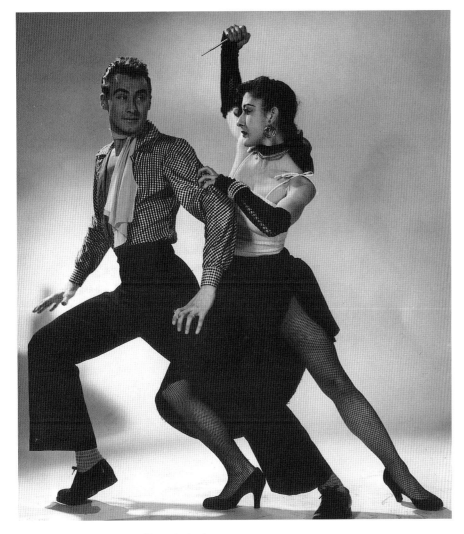

Arnold Spohr and Eva von Gencsy in an apache number for the Winnipeg Ballet, about 1950. Eva von Gencsy joined the company in 1948, shortly after arriving in Canada as a refugee from Eastern Europe. She later became artistic director of Les Ballets Jazz in Montreal. (Phillips-Gutkin photograph)

Facing page: Winnipeg Ballet principals Jean McKenzie, later founding director of the company school, and Arnold Spohr, for 30 years the company's artistic director, in their days as a popular performing partnership, about 1950. (Phillips-Gutkin photograph)

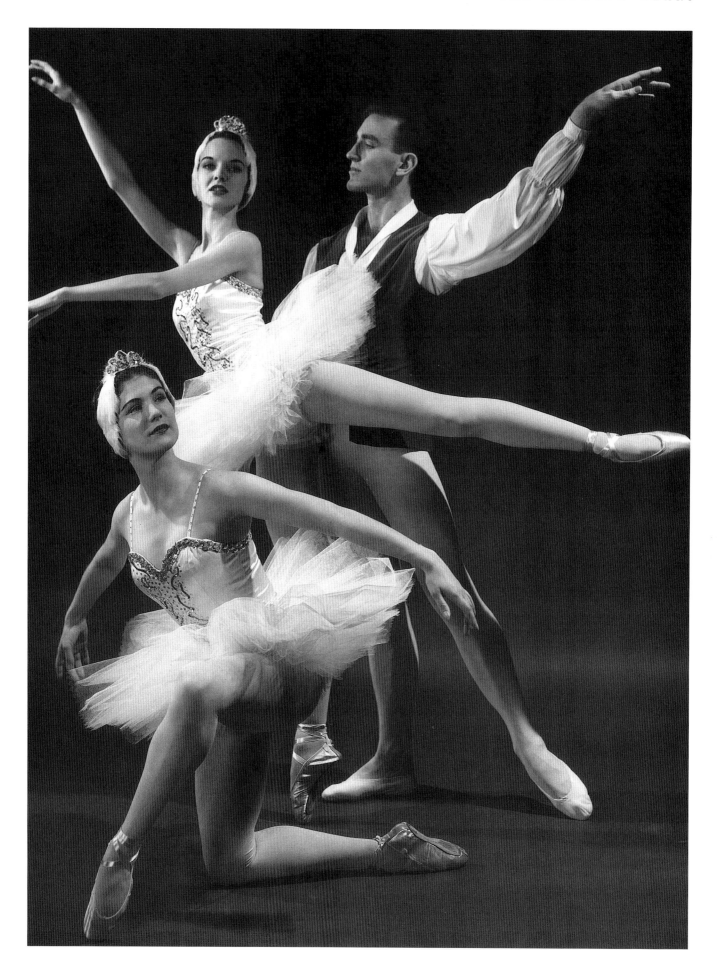

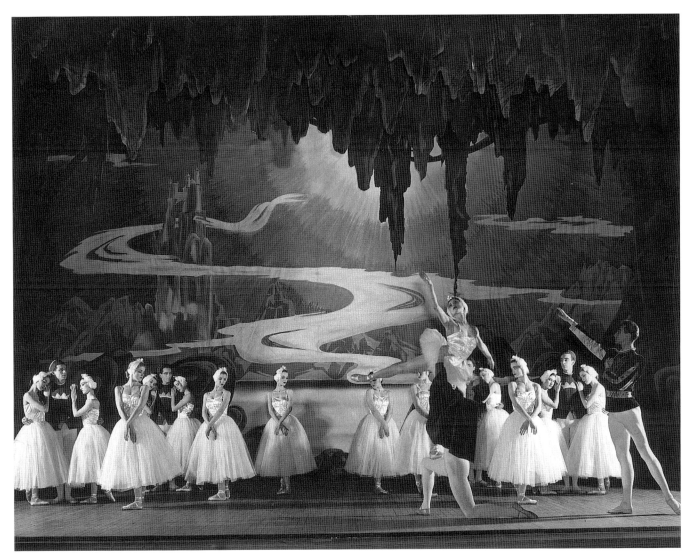

Facing page: The Royal Winnipeg Ballet carried extracts from *Swan Lake* in a variety of versions prior to its acquisition of the full Galina Yordanova production in 1987. This mid-1950s photo shows (*left to right*) Marsha Wardall, Marilyn Young and Brendon Fitzgerald in Mary Skeaping's staging of the Act I *pas de trois.* (Phillips-Gutkin photograph)

Arnold Spohr and Eva von Gencsy in the Winnipeg Ballet's 1952 production of *Swan Lake, Act II,* staged "after Petipa." Eva von Gencsy's White Swan was regarded as one of her finest roles. (Phillips-Gutkin photograph)

Shadow on the Prairie, made by Gweneth
Lloyd for the Winnipeg Ballet, was
welcomed as "a Canadian work of major
stature" at its 1952 premiere. A tragic
story of a homesick immigrant, it was the
first ballet filmed by the National Film
Board. Carlu Carter, as the central figure,
appears here with Gordon Wales.
(Courtesy Gweneth Lloyd)

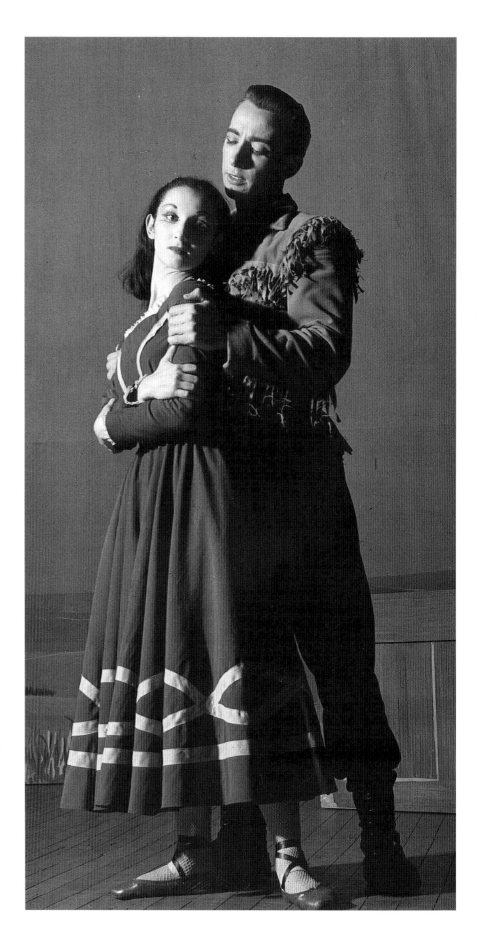

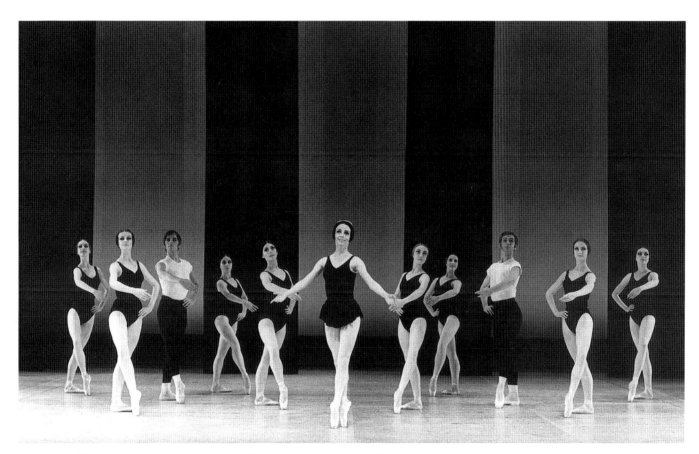

Aimez-vous Bach? grows from a dance class to a large ensemble work, closing with a jive-and-twist sequence to Bach's *D Minor Toccata and Fugue.* Made in 1962, the work was mounted on the Royal Winnipeg Ballet in 1964, the year it won a gold star for choreographer Brian Macdonald at the Paris International Dance Festival. (Martha Swope photograph)

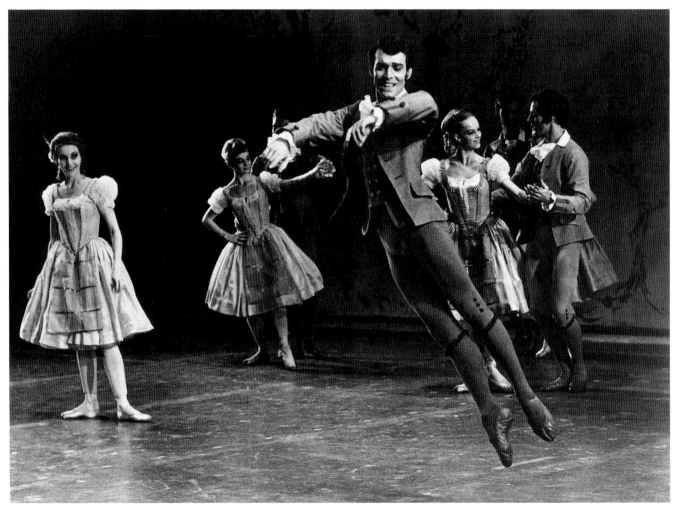

U.S. choreographer Eliot Feld's *Meadow
Lark,* a sunlit gambol for six couples, was
created for the Royal Winnipeg Ballet in
1968. It was one of four works, presented
on a single bill, that provoked critic Clive
Barnes to enthuse about the RWB's
"prairie freshness." Richard Rutherford
danced the original male lead. (Martha
Swope photograph)

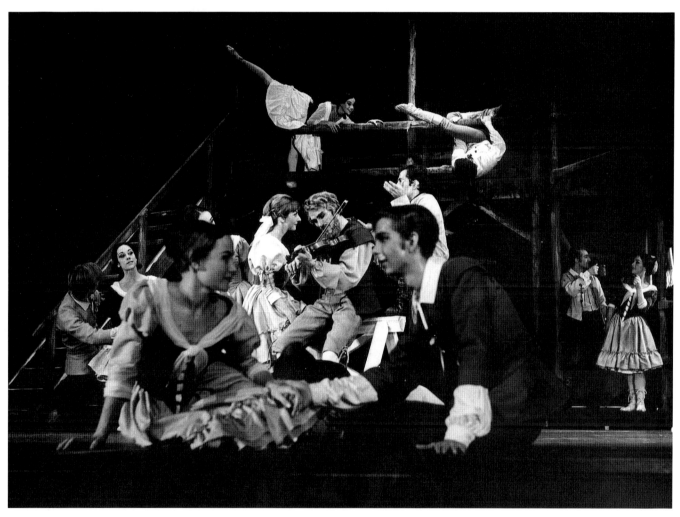

Brian Macdonald's rendering of the traditional legend of *Rose Latulippe,* claimed as the first full-length ballet on a Canadian theme, was the Royal Winnipeg Ballet's contribution to the nation's centennial festivities. It was introduced at the Stratford Festival in 1966. (Douglas Spillane photograph, courtesy Royal Winnipeg Ballet)

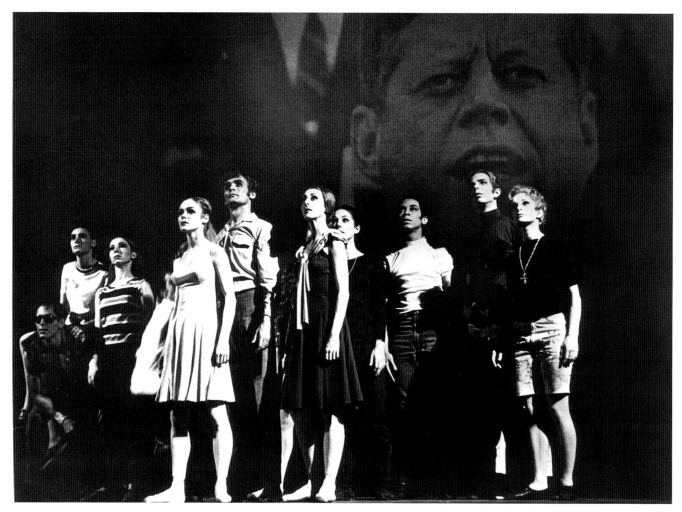

Inspired by lines from a poem on the death of John F. Kennedy, Brian Macdonald's *While the Spider Slept* was made for the Royal Swedish Ballet in 1965. Mounted on the Royal Winnipeg Ballet the following year, it was greeted as "a very subtle and serious work of conscience and of art." (Peter Garrick photograph)

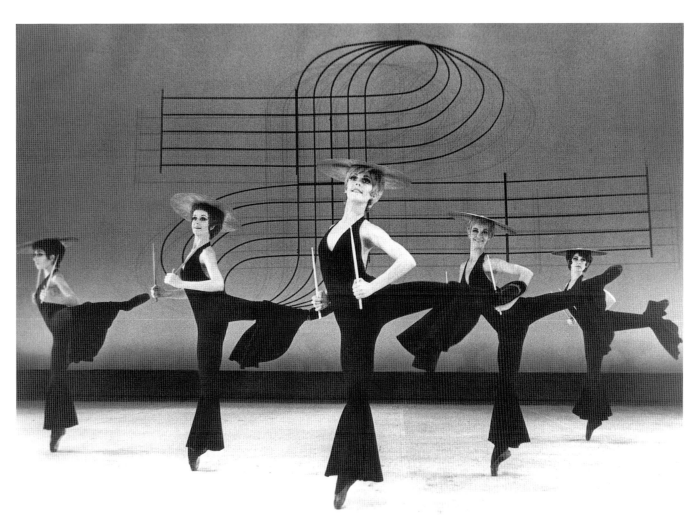

The Winnipeg Ballet's first principal male dancer, Paddy Stone, became a prominent light-entertainment and TV choreographer in England. He returned to Canada in 1969 to mount his *Variations on Strike Up the Band* for the Royal Winnipeg Ballet. (Martha Swope photograph)

Geneviève Salbaing, later one of the co-founders of Les Ballets Jazz, performed with Les Ballets Chiriaeff in the early 1950s. She is shown here in a production for the TV series *L'Heure du concert.* (Henri Paul photograph, courtesy Geneviève Salbaing)

Facing page: Margaret Mercier and Eric Hyrst are shown in the Black Swan pas de deux from Hyrst's setting of *Swan Lake, Act II* for Les Grands Ballets Canadiens, in the 1959–60 season. (Gaby photograph, courtesy Les Grands Ballets Canadiens)

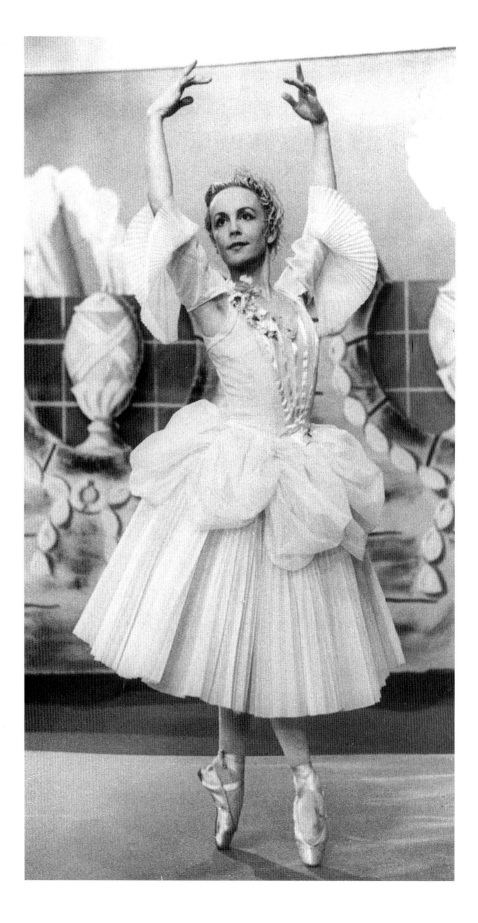

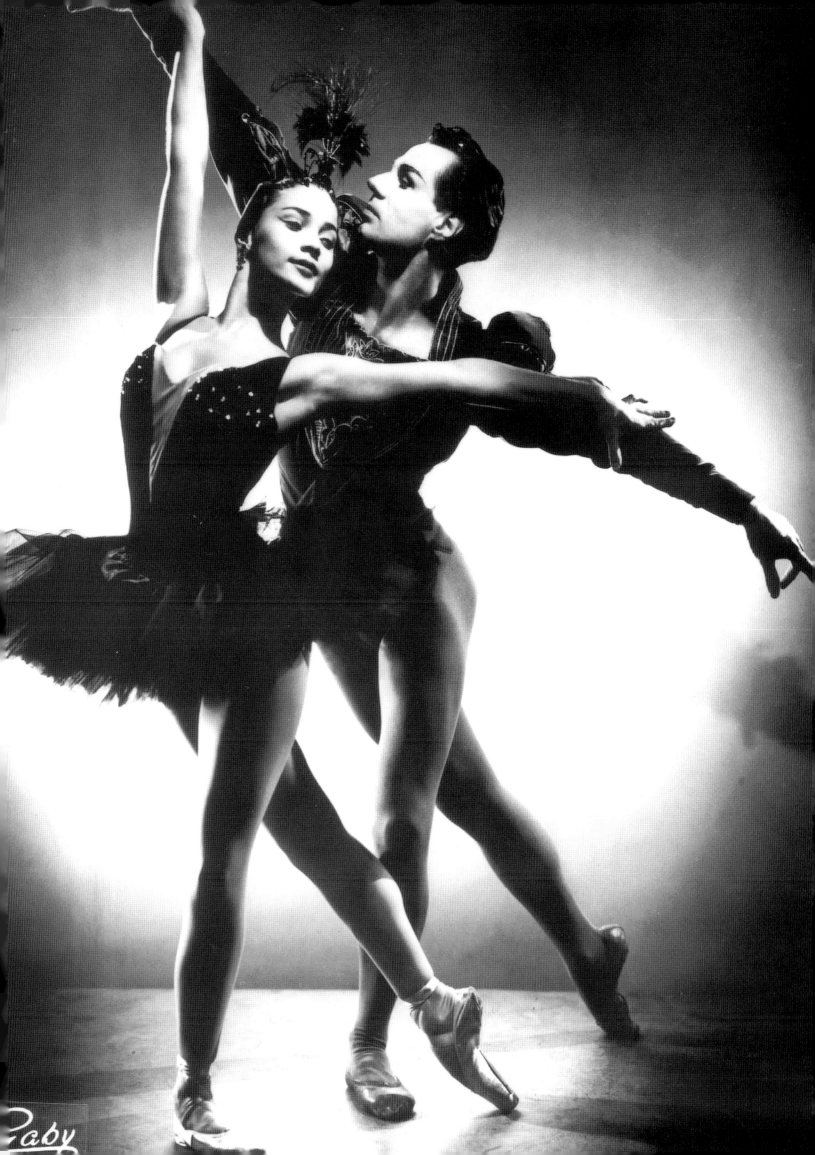

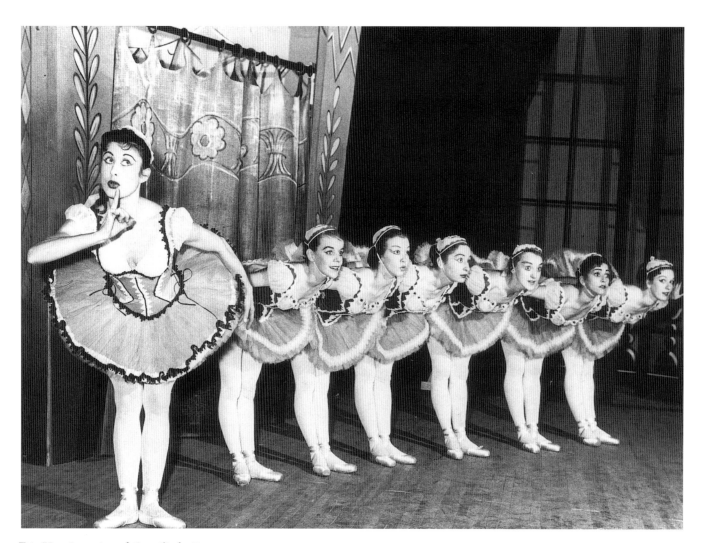

Eric Hyrst's staging of *Coppélia* for Les
Grands Ballets Canadiens was first
produced for *L'Heure du concert* in 1956.
It entered the company's live-stage
repertoire in 1958, with Eva von Gencsy
in the lead. (Courtesy Les Grands Ballets
Canadiens)

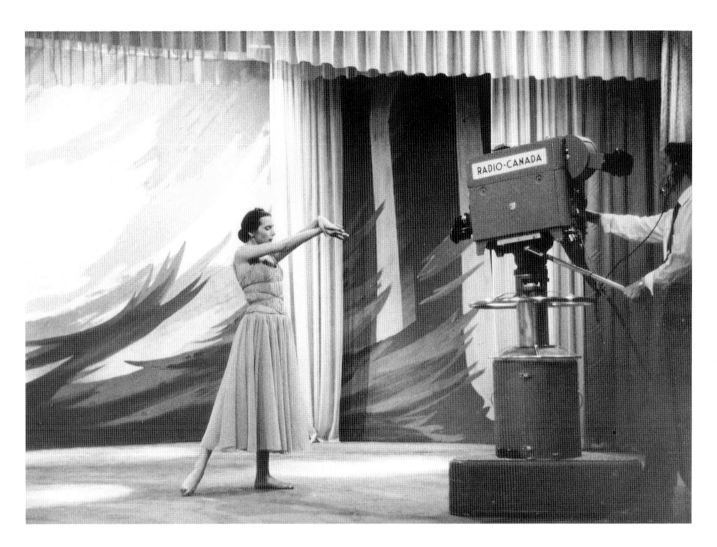

Ludmilla Chiriaeff leads Les Ballets
Chiriaeff in Eric Hyrst's *Variations sur un
thème de Haydn* for the television series
L'Heure du concert in May 1955. (Henri
Paul photograph, courtesy Ludmilla
Chiriaeff)

Ludmilla Chiriaeff and Eric Hyrst with
the corps de ballet of Les Grands Ballets
Canadiens perform her staging of *Les
Noces* (first televised on *L'Heure du
concert*) at its first live performance at the
Festival de Montreal in September 1956.
(Courtesy Les Grands Ballets Canadiens)

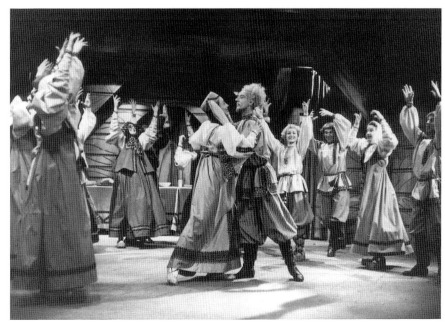

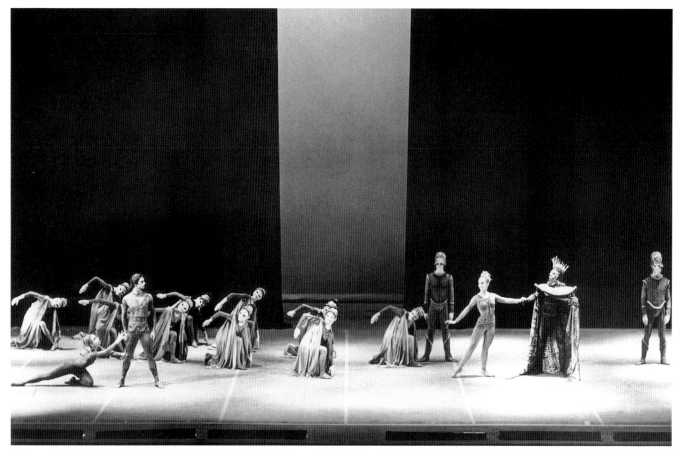

Brydon Paige made his version of the
Euripides play *Medea* for Les Grands
Ballets in 1962, to a commissioned
electronic score by Georges Savaria. Lead
performers here are Veronique Landory,
Armando Jorge, Nicole Vachon and Bill
Thompson. (Henry Koro photograph,
courtesy Les Grands Ballets Canadiens)

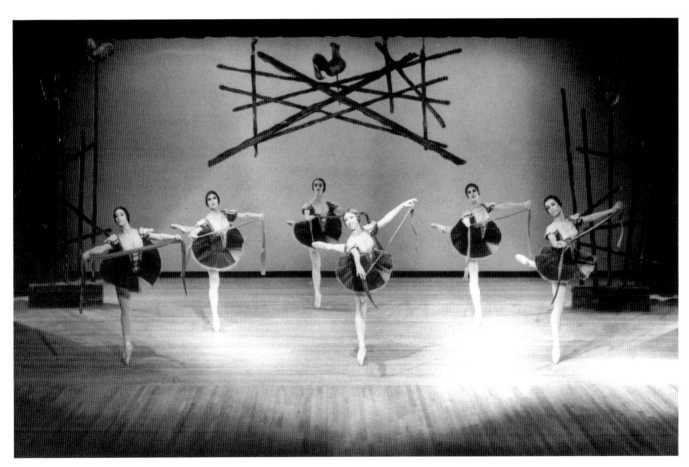

Ludmilla Chiriaeff's *Canadiana* entered the repertoire of Les Grands Ballets Canadiens in the 1960–61 season. Shown here is Andrée Millaire (*centre*), with Linda Stearns (*extreme right*), later to become involved in the company's direction. (Courtesy Les Grands Ballets Canadiens)

Modern Dance

AMERICAN MODERNISM CATCHES ON

In the years following the Second World War, control over what Canadians saw and thought would swing slowly across the Atlantic, away from Europe and into the United States. But the process was by no means instantaneous. The new movements in art that were occurring below the border—in dance in particular—were slow to catch on in Canada.

In modern dance, the European influence in the immediate postwar years was principally Wigman-style German expressionism, represented at the ballet festivals by the Sorel company, the Neo-Dance Theatre of Toronto (1949), the New Dance Theatre (1950 and 1952) and the Montreal Modern Dance Company (1954). The Neo-Dance Theatre and the New Dance Theatre were connected through choreographer-teacher Nancy Lima Dent, who had studied with Volkoff and Leese before going to the U.S. for studies with Doris Humphrey and the Wigman disciple Hanya Holm. Dent also tried Graham, but found its technical formula too restricting. She began to choreograph in 1946, at the age of 27, and became co-director—along with another expressionist choreographer, Cynthia Barrett—of the newly formed Neo-Dance Theatre. However, by the time they appeared at the 1949 festival, there had been disagreements over artistic policy and Dent had left.

She established the New Dance Theatre soon after. Her first work was a mime-and-movement response to a poem about the atom bomb and the dangers of uranium. *That We May Live* dealt with the sufferings of Slavic and Jewish peoples in Czarist Russia and their liberation through emigration to Canada. *Heroes of Our Time*, seen at the 1952 festival, was a study in juvenile delinquency.

According to Herbert Whittaker, in *DanceMagazine*, the work used "comparatively little ballet and a great deal of dramatic mime." The conservatives raised the usual protest at this, though Whittaker himself defended the right of groups like Dent's to a place in the festival. "It was a relief to find," he wrote, "in contrast to teacher-pupil groups paying tribute to the past, an experimental company for which choreography is a collective thing. And, one which is spurred on by a dominant idea. People who couldn't see the dancing for the idea applauded quite blissfully at other groups which danced without even the shadow of an idea."

The debate that was to divide the traditionalists and the innovators for the next three decades was warming up.

The New Dance Theatre's activities ended when Dent moved to Sudbury in 1955, but she continued to create, later returning to Toronto and setting up the Nancy Lima Dent Dance Company.

In Montreal, meanwhile, the modernist torch was taken up by Yone Kvietys, a

Lithuanian who had studied in the Wigman style and at the Laban school in Hamburg before emigrating to Canada in 1948. She danced briefly with the Volkoff company, then moved to Montreal, where the Montreal Modern Dance Company gave its first full-length concert in January 1954. Kvietys was listed as artistic director, but equal choreographic credit was given to Biroute Nagys, from Germany, and Alexander MacDougall, a Montrealer (ex-Leese, ex-Sorel) who had formerly been a soloist with the Ballet Jooss in Europe. The company appeared at the 1954 ballet festival, dancing two works credited jointly to Kvietys and Nagys.

The company was short-lived, but in 1959 Kvietys made contact in Toronto with Nancy Lima Dent, Ruth (Tutti) Lau (another German immigrant) and Bianca Rogge, a Latvian. Rogge, who studied and taught at the Wigman school in Berlin in the 1930s, had moved to Canada in 1956. Her dancing was called, variously, "German impressionistic," "modern" and "interpretive"; masks featured prominently in her work.

These four women, calling themselves Contemporary Choreographers of Toronto, mounted a "festival" evening of modern dance in February 1960—the first time a group of modern dancers had staged a joint concert in Canada.

"Ultimately," said the advance publicity, "it is hoped that a Canadian modern dance company will be formed, composed of the best modern dancers in Canada and as a vehicle for Canadian and American contemporary choreographers." The reference to the need for a vehicle for Canadian and *American* choreographers underlined the new creative reality. The vital forces in European modern dance were at a low ebb. America was where the modernist action was, and it is an irony of the history of dancing in Canada that while the earliest beginnings of its modernist school were to be found in the country's European roots, the impetus for its development—the impetus that would push idea, or ideal, into reality—was the example of what was happening in America. It was a lasting transference of influence.

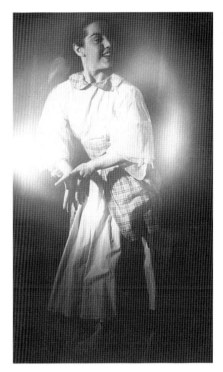

Nancy Lima Dent in Earl Robinson's Lonesome Train, *for the New Dance Theatre in 1950. "There is not too much praise I can bestow upon the brilliant New Dance Theatre," said Anatole Chujoy of* Dance News *after the 1950 Ballet Festival. "I found their performance to be stimulating in the highest artistic sense." (Nancy Lima Dent Collection, Dance Collection Danse, Toronto)*

———

The story of the evolution of modern dance in North America in this century has been, throughout, a story of revolution—the revolution of the early barefoot dancers against the traditions of ballet, the revolution of Graham's descendants against the psychological-expressive and the mythic-theatrical in favour of pure movement. But by the 1950s dance itself was only part of a larger revolution that had grown out of the global anxieties of the time, as artists, responding to a society in which the comfortable predictability of tradition was consistently undermined by chance, rejected meaning in a manner that echoed the audacious nihilism of the Dadaists and the retreat by Europe's surrealists into the subconscious.

Sartre's existentialism and Ionesco's theatre of the absurd had led to Beckett's *Waiting for Godot*. In 1952, the year that *Godot* appeared, John Cage staged the first multidisciplinary "happening," putting the world on notice that former concepts of acceptability in performance no longer held. His collaborator, Merce Cunningham, a defector from the Graham camp, tossed aside conventional notions of meaning and declared that movement justified itself in its very existence. "The logic of one event coming as responsive to another seems inadequate now," he wrote. Change was on its way. And dancing would never be the same.

In the summer of 1961, composer Pierre Mercure organized a Modern Music Week in Montreal. Modernism in Montreal was having a tough time of it; Mercure, encouraged and excited by his frequent contacts with music's avant-garde in New York, wanted to demystify the performing arts.

In attendance were the leading lights of European new music, Karlheinz Stockhausen, Mauricio Kagel, Christiann Wolff and Iannis Xenakis, and from New York, John Cage, Merce Cunningham, performance artist Yoko Ono and choreographer Alwin Nikolais, an innovator in the area of mixed media. The event predated by a year the first interdisciplinary presentations by New York's influential Judson Church group.

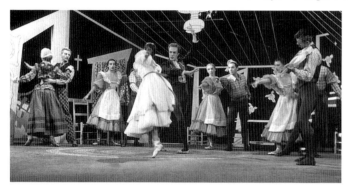

In Françoise Sullivan's version of Rose Latulipe *[sic] for* CBC *Radio-Canada's* Allo Toronto . . . Ici Montréal TV *program in 1953, Heino Heiden plays the Devil, Roland Boisvenu is the Violinist and Lise Gagné is Rose. (Courtesy Françoise Sullivan)*

The week's principal significance for dance in Montreal was that it brought Jeanne Renaud back into the fold. After her involvement with *les automatistes* in the 1940s, she had settled in Paris, where she had made dance experiments with the colony of expatriate Montreal artists. Mercure wrote some of his earliest experimental music for her performances, with composer Gabriel Charpentier and Mercure's cello-playing wife Monique in the orchestra; painter Jean-Pierre Riopelle decorated the set with moving projections he created by plucking hairs from his head and placing them on slides to allow the heat of the projection lamp to curl the hair.

But by the time Renaud returned to Montreal in the mid-1950s, she had tired of dance and did not perform again until Françoise Riopelle (another signatory to *refus global*, and herself recently returned from Paris) asked her to deputize for an injured dancer at Mercure's Modern Music Week.

The experience—particularly its reaffirmation of the surrealist and Dadaist principles that had been so important to *les automatistes*—fanned the embers. Soon, Renaud and Riopelle launched the Modern Dance Group of Montreal, but critics said their work, heavily influenced by the unemotional geometrics favoured by the visual artists of the time, lacked warmth, and their audiences were small.

It needed the enthusiasm of a ballet dancer, Vincent Warren, a principal with Les Grands Ballets Canadiens, to push these tentative beginnings towards true professionalism. Warren, always eager for anything that might expand his own horizons, worked regularly with Renaud and Riopelle, and in 1965 he introduced them to another dancer from Les Grands, Peter Boneham. Boneham had worked with Warren in New York in 1960, and through Warren's close friendship with the poet Frank O'Hara he had become involved with New York's artistic avant-garde, particularly the dance experimenters.

Boneham and Renaud clicked immediately, and he agreed to perform with her in a show called Expressions 65. Shortly after, he suggested she form a performing company, and it was launched in 1966 as Le Groupe de la Place Royale—a title intended to signify a coming-together of artists, rather than simply a troupe of dancers. That year, Le Groupe became the first modern-dance company to receive a grant from the Canada Council: a token $3,500, regarded, in the words of council director Peter Dwyer, as "a calculated risk."

In 1961, the year Pierre Mercure's Modern Music Week showed Montreal what the music and dance avant-garde of New York was up to, a similar event was held in Vancouver—a Festival of the Contemporary Arts, organized by B. C. Binning, head of fine arts at the University of British Columbia. The festival ran annually for a decade, and brought to the city a range of American innovators in all disciplines—among them Cunningham and one of the pioneers of dance "happenings," Ann Halprin. By 1964 the Vancouver community was feeling sufficiently encouraged to begin to mount experimental events of its own under the festival umbrella.

Early in 1963, the first modern dance festival involving dancers from across Canada was held in Toronto. Walter Sorell in *DanceMagazine* described it as an effort to create a better understanding in Canada of the barefoot, tutu-less dancer. Featured alongside three of the 1960-festival originals (Kvietys, Rogge and Lau) were Biroute Nagys, from Montreal, Freda Crisp, from Hamilton, Ontario, and Norbert Vesak, from Vancouver. Sorell had reservations about what he saw, but he wrote: "Under all its groping, flailing and moments of fulfilment, this festival seemed determined to find the way to the future."

The future, as it happened, was close at hand.

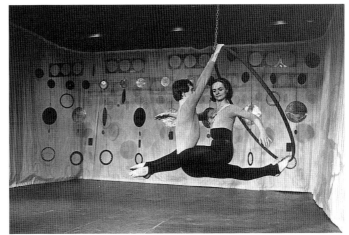

Jeanne Renaud and Peter Boneham, co-founders of Le Groupe de la Place Royale, in Rideau, *at Expressions 65, the 1965 production that brought them together. The mobile set (by Françoise Sullivan) was struck by the dancers to provide the sonic accompaniment for the piece. (Marc-André Gagné photograph, courtesy Françoise Sullivan)*

A DIFFERENT FOOTING: *Toronto Dance Theatre*

The Toronto Dance Theatre had its origins, according to one of its founders, on top of a Liverpool bus.

It was 1967. David Earle and Peter Randazzo had been involved in the proposed launching of a Graham-based company in England, the London Contemporary Dance Theatre. The experience had been traumatic—physical violence had broken out in connection with a programme marking the opening of a new cathedral in Liverpool—and as Randazzo recalls it: "We were on one of those red buses, just David and me, at the front of the bus, on the top. I said: 'Hey, David, why don't we start a dance company?' Without thinking, he said: 'Sure. What'll we call it?' I said: 'Toronto Dance Theatre.' End of conversation."

David Earle was born in Toronto in 1940. He spent 11 years as a child performing Greek myths and Indian legends with the Toronto Children's Theatre, fell in love with dance when he saw the Bolshoi Ballet on a visit to Toronto's Maple Leaf Gardens, and at the age of 20 enrolled at the newly launched National Ballet School.

During his four years at the school he danced with modernist choreographer Yone Kvietys, and in the summer of 1963, inspired by his experiences as a performer at the Toronto modern dance festival that spring, he attended the Connecticut College summer dance course in New London. One of his teachers was

Martha Graham. She made a deep impression, and the following year he enrolled at the Graham school in New York. Among his colleagues were James Cunningham, another Toronto Children's Theatre alumnus who later founded a company in the U.S., and Toronto-born Patricia Beatty.

There was often talk among the Canadians at the Graham studio about the possibility of opening a Graham-based school in Toronto, and in 1965 Beatty went to Toronto to demonstrate for a series of Graham classes at the National Ballet School. Soon, Beatty had a studio of her own—"I made it as beautiful as I could, copied Martha, a brown barre . . . I put beautiful things up. It looked thoughtful"—and in December 1967, while Earle and Randazzo were still thinking about the idea of a Toronto Dance Theatre, she launched the New Dance Group of Canada.

For the opening show, Beatty did a dance called *Momentum*, based on *Macbeth*, to music by Ann Southam, and there were two guest choreographers: Cynthia Barrett, an early collaborator with Nancy Lima Dent in the Neo-Dance Theatre; and Randazzo, a principal with the Graham company, who was in town with Earle on a visit. Randazzo's work, *Fragments*, was his first venture into choreography and was danced by himself, Earle and Beatty. Its presentation was one of the few occasions on which the three co-founders of the Toronto Dance Theatre ever appeared on stage together.

In the Toronto *Telegram*, Ralph Hicklin called the appearance of the new company "an occasion—as much an occasion as, say, the National Ballet's first performance of *Romeo and Juliet*."

"To come upon such stylish cohesion in any locally-managed theatre presentation is unusual," wrote Nathan Cohen, in the Toronto *Star*. "To discover it in a modern . . . dance recital is unprecedented." He concluded: "Modern dance has been a long time coming to Toronto. There have been some attempts . . . they failed to take hold, usually with good reason. Now surely is a more favourable time."

He was a little ahead of himself.

After the spring presentation in Toronto, Earle returned to London, serving briefly as artistic director of the London Contemporary Dance Theatre, and Randazzo returned to the Graham company. Neither was happy; what they wanted was a company of their own, and that fall they returned to Toronto and persuaded John Sime, founder of Toronto's Three Schools of Arts, to finance its creation. A matter of days before they were due to sign the contract with Sime, Earle and Randazzo were approached by Beatty. She proposed they join forces. They agreed, and the Toronto Dance Theatre made its debut in December 1968.

Its connection with the Martha Graham tradition has been a source of much

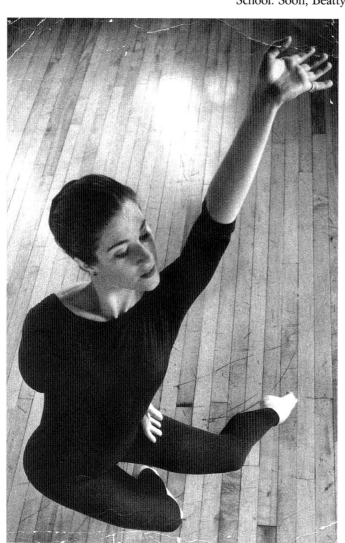

Patricia Beatty, co-founder of Toronto Dance Theatre, was raised to be a lawyer but rebelled and turned to dance, studying for five years at the Martha Graham school in New York. She is seen here shortly after her return to Canada in 1965, at work in her first studio in Toronto. (Courtesy Patricia Beatty)

confusion because of the trio's admiration for the Graham style and their personal links with her company. The three founders subsequently claimed they never set out to create a mini-Graham company. What they took from Graham was her movement technique, but their choreographic style, they insisted, was their own. Earle's language of movement, in its use of symbolism and its emphasis on myth, is the closest to Graham's own, though his own view is that his work is more narrative, less abstract and "less masculine" than Graham's. Beatty's idiom shares a dynamic force with Graham, but it has about it what Earle calls "humane abstraction" (Beatty thinks it has just enough form for her audiences to make contact with what she wants to say). Randazzo's style is a kind of danced abstract expressionism, rarely literal or narrative, but more an interaction of energies, expressed in a highly poetic manner.

In the early years the company's associations with New York modernism attracted an arts-community audience, but general public understanding was hard to come by. Beatty believes the challenges wore the three of them out. "I think it aged us. I think there would be more dances, and the three of us would be dancing better, if we had had someone who knew what to do with a modern dance company. But how was anyone supposed to know? We just made it up. And when you don't know, you use up so much energy."

Susan Macpherson, one of the earliest company members (ex-Kvietys, ex-Graham school), remembers those first years as an optimistic, idealistic time, everyone working for $40 a week. It was like a family; and when, after three or four years, the first core group of dancers decided to move on, the founders were shocked. "It felt like treason just to say you were leaving," says Keith Urban, who danced in the first company and stayed for four years. But it wasn't just a matter of departing dancers. Audiences, never numerous, had begun to desert the company as well.

A HANDFUL OF VISIONARIES ACROSS THE WEST

Across western Canada, the story of the development of modern dance is—like the story of the early years of ballet in Canada—the story of a handful of visionaries, mostly women, who struggled against great odds to scratch into inhospitable ground enough of a space to give the seed of modernism a chance to grow.

One of the earliest of the modernist professionals in Western Canada was Rachel Browne, who did not start out as a modernist at all, but went on to found what was to become Canada's oldest professional modern dance company, Winnipeg's Contemporary Dancers. Browne, born in Philadelphia, was one of a group imported by Benjamin Harkarvy when he took over artistic directorship of the Royal Winnipeg Ballet in 1957.

Her swing from ballet to modern dance happened only gradually. She spent several summers studying Graham, Limón and Cunningham techniques in New York, began to choreograph on her students, and launched the company in 1964 as an *ad hoc* group at the University of Manitoba. Over the years she supplemented her own choreography with a steady stream of guest works from a range of U.S. modernists and many of the driving forces of new Canadian dance.

The company always survived by extensive touring to small towns, and the intense and committed Browne evolved a programming philosophy that in some ways mirrored the demands for accessibility laid down by the founders of the RWB itself, leavened by what she once called "a humanism about our work, a conscious desire to communicate emotion and excitement to our audience, helping to improve the quality of life in all those two-by-four towns that haven't had contact with modern dance before."

In Vancouver, some of the earliest modern dance teaching in the city came from the sisters Gertrud and Magda Hanova. Born in Bohemia in the early part of the century, they trained in Germany in the Wigman style and in Dalcroze gymnastics, and settled in Vancouver in the late 1950s.

Professional modern dance did not arrive in Vancouver until the late 1960s. The first individual to establish a professional modern dance company in Vancouver was Paula Ross, a former ballet student who had gypsied around the U.S. and Canada as a nightclub dancer and chorus-girl before returning to Vancouver in the early 1960s. She launched an informal performing group in 1965, but did not receive government funding until 1974. A driven and emotional woman, Ross evolved a choreographic style she called "visual poetry," rooted in a raw, emotional expressiveness. Of partly native Indian ancestry, she attempts, she once explained, to express "a universal tribal metaphor." She won the Chalmers choreographic award in 1977. Her company suspended operations in 1987, but during its existence she was widely regarded as the authentic choreographic voice of the popular image of the West Coast—romantic, unhurried, idiosyncratic, hedonistic.

One of the first persons to teach an organized modern dance technique on the West Coast was Norbert Vesak, the sole West Coast participant in the 1963 festival in Toronto. Born in British Columbia in 1936, Vesak trained in both modern dance and classical ballet, and studied at Jacob's Pillow, in London and in New York before returning to Vancouver in the 1960s and becoming involved in 1964 in an abortive attempt to launch a crossover ballet-and-modern company with ballet teacher and choreographer Joy Camden.

By this time, the city was welcoming a range of U.S. dance modernists, introduced principally by the universities—Helen Goodwin at the University of British Columbia (her own experimental group, TheCo, founded in 1964, featured prominently in the annual modernist festivals) and Iris Garland, in the process of launching the dance programme at Simon Fraser University.

By 1968 Vesak was presenting concerts using his students; in the spring of 1970 he launched Western Dance Theatre, with a guest appearance by Lynn Seymour, dancing Kenneth MacMillan's *Solitaire*. In its first season the company rode a wave of public optimism and enthusiasm, but financial problems, administrative and personnel troubles and negative press response led to the company's abrupt closure midway through its second season.

Almost immediately, Vesak was invited by Arnold Spohr to make *The Ecstasy of Rita Joe* for the Royal Winnipeg Ballet.

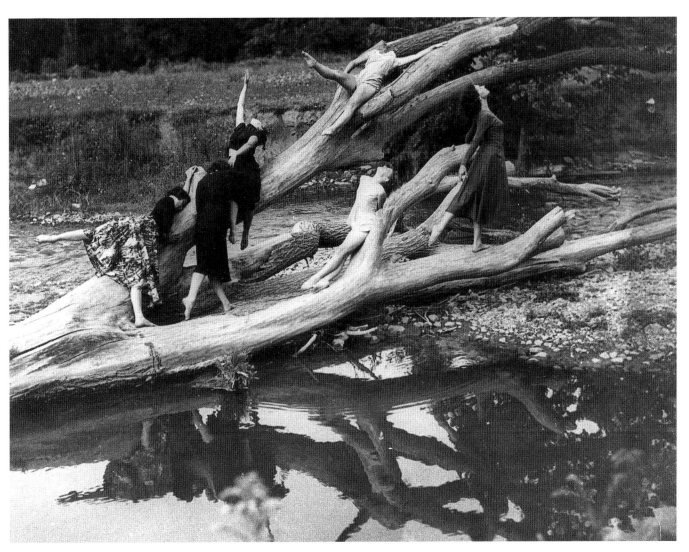

Members of Nancy Lima Dent's New Dance Theatre, located in Toronto, in the 1950s. (Courtesy Nancy Lima Dent)

Overleaf: Alexander MacDougall, Yone Kvietys and Biroute Nagys (*prostrate*) in *Dark Vision,* a work created jointly by Kvietys and Nagys for the first performance of the Montreal Modern Dance Company in 1954. (I. Wachnianyn photograph, courtesy Alexander MacDougall)

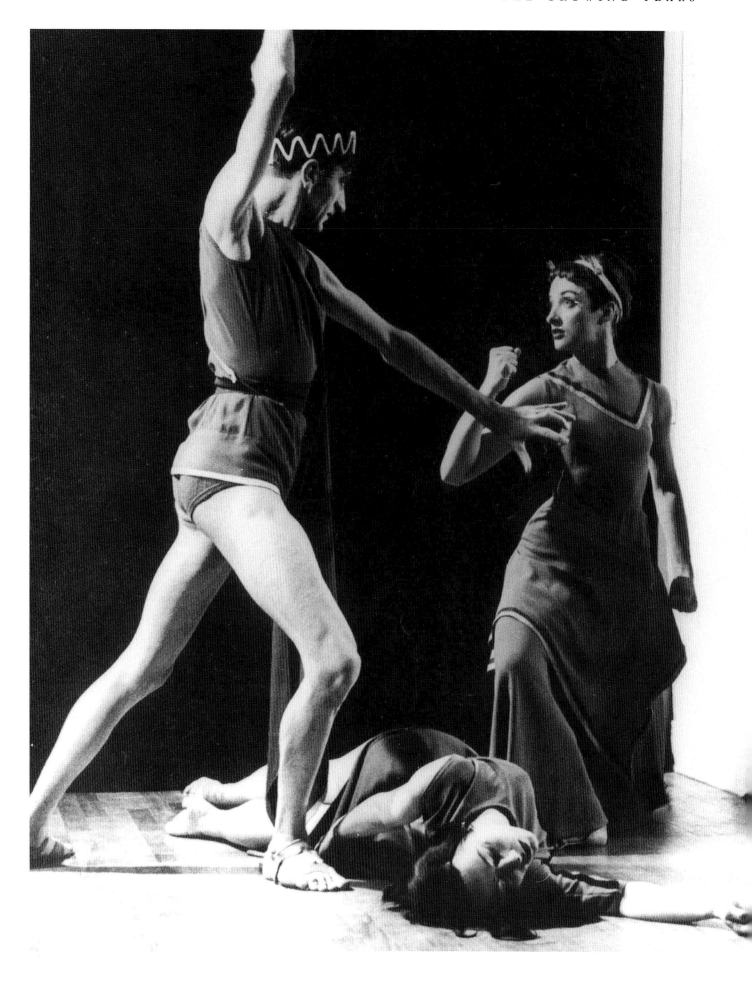

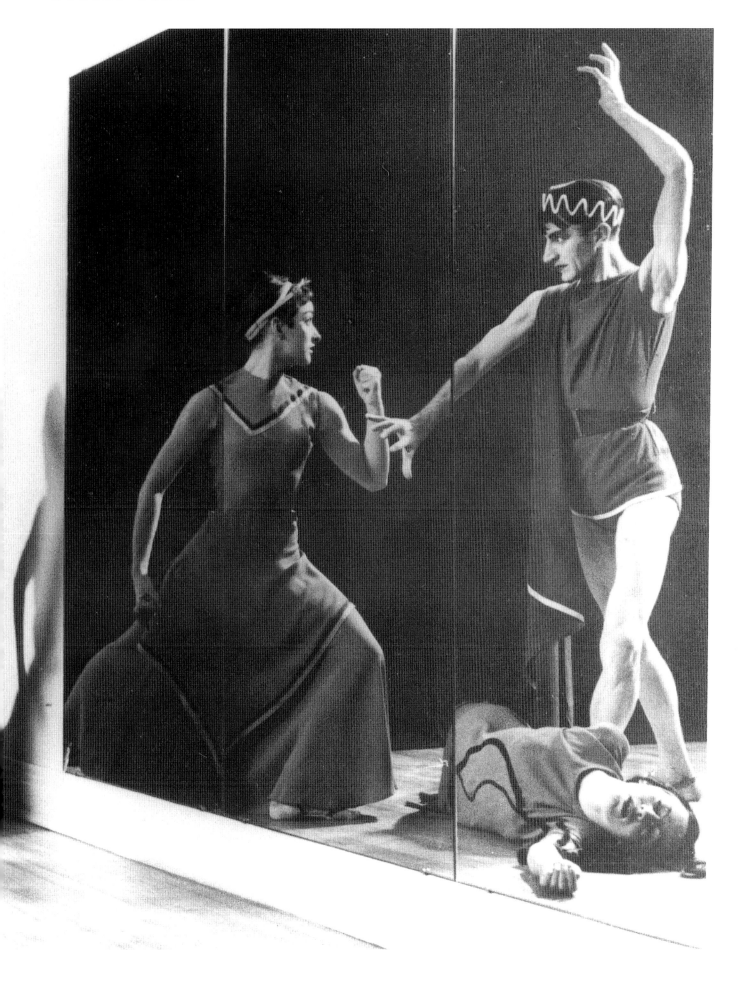

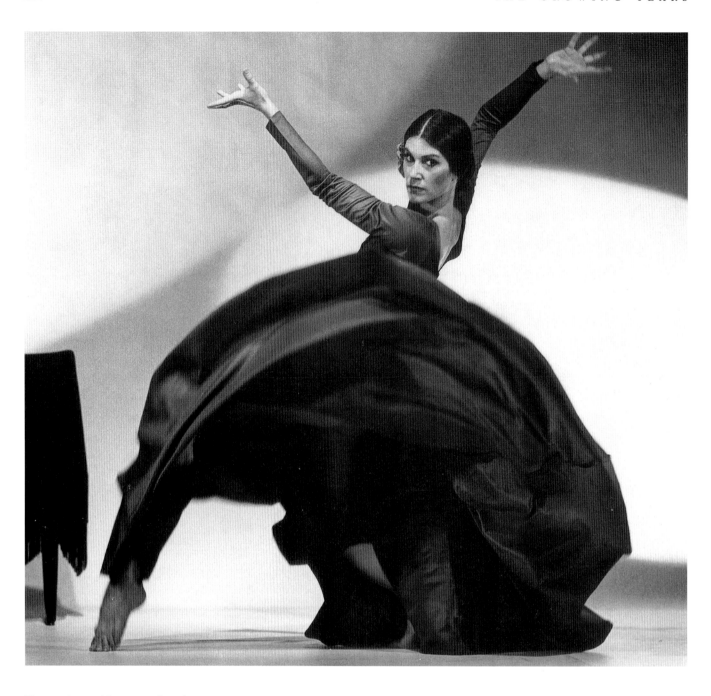

Toronto Dance Theatre co-founder
Patricia Beatty in her 1979 work, *Lessons
in Another Language,* which set the bold
and flamboyant movement of Spanish
dance against the casual work-movement
of a stage hand. (Andrew Oxenham
photograph)

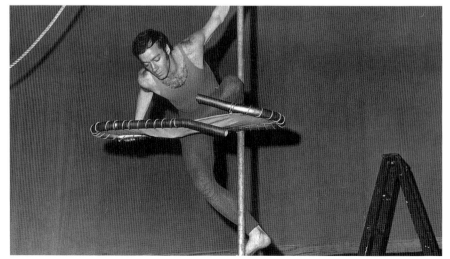

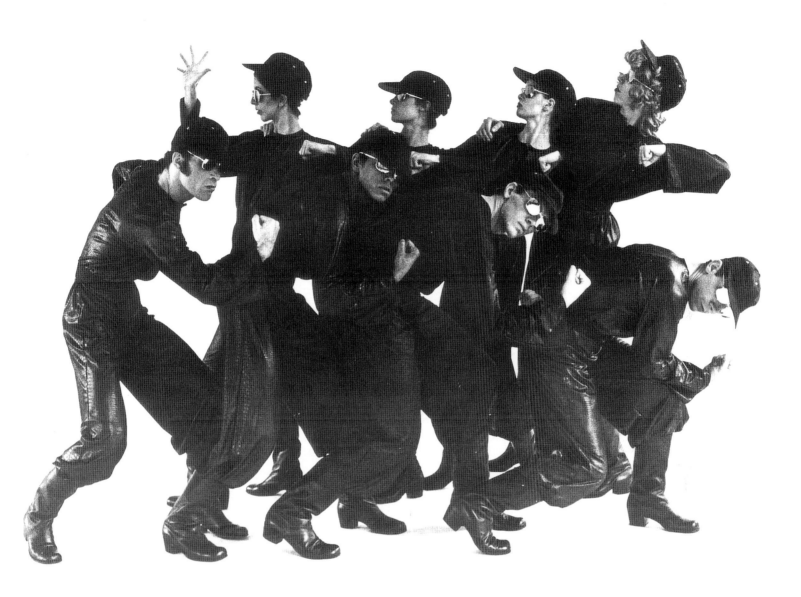

Facing page, bottom: Patricia Beatty's *Against Sleep,* made in 1968, was one of the earliest works in the Toronto Dance Theatre repertoire. Its theme is the temptation of suicide, with a mysterious Guest (David Earle in this still from a CBC performance) dominating a Woman's anxiety-ridden night. (CBC photograph, courtesy Patricia Beatty)

Peter Randazzo's satire on dance and society, *A Simple Melody,* made for Toronto Dance Theatre in 1977, "was like some incredible combination of Doris Humphrey at the Greek Theatre and a 1920s *Saturday Evening Post* ad for bottled water," said the *Ottawa Review,* "and it brought the house down." (David Davis photograph)

U.S. modernist Norman Walker's *Three Psalms,* mounted on Winnipeg's Contemporary Dancers in 1969, opened with a duet in which the dancers wore transparent material that Walker said was designed "to keep those parts of the body which cannot be choreographed under control." Pictured are Leslie Dillingham and William Holahan. (Courtesy Contemporary Dancers)

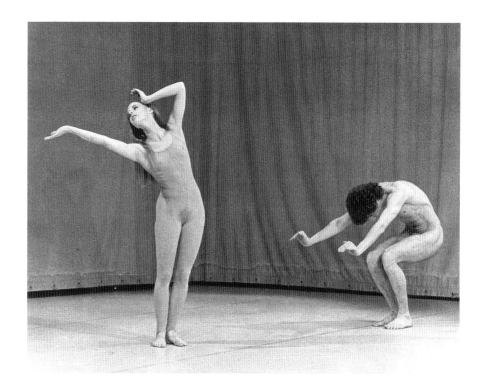

Rachel Browne made her solo, *Cameo,* for Winnipeg's Contemporary Dancers in 1965, shortly after the company was founded under her artistic directorship, and performed it for a week's run at Expo 67 in Montreal. (Andrew Oxenham photograph)

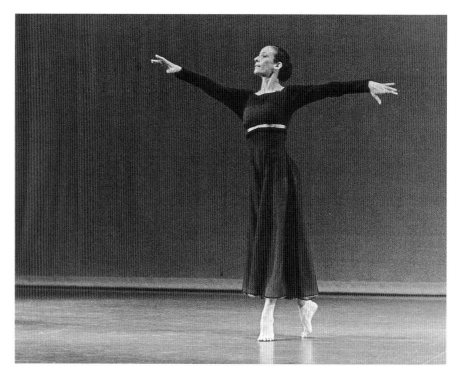

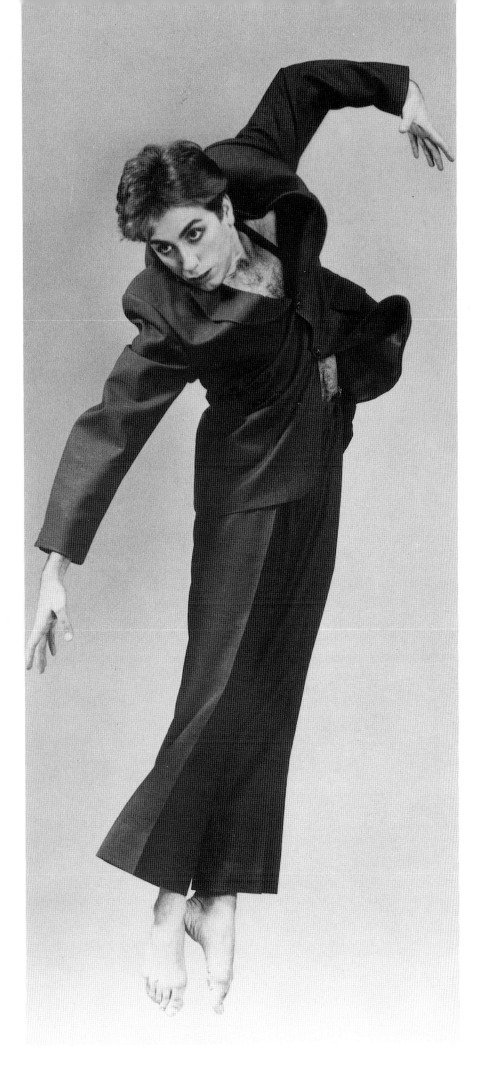

Tedd Robinson, subsequently artistic director of Winnipeg's Contemporary Dancers, in a 1978 photograph from the company's production of Karen Jamieson's *Snakes and Ladders.* At that time, the company was still operating under artistic director Rachel Browne as a repertory modern dance company showcasing Canadian and U.S. choreographers. (David Cooper photograph)

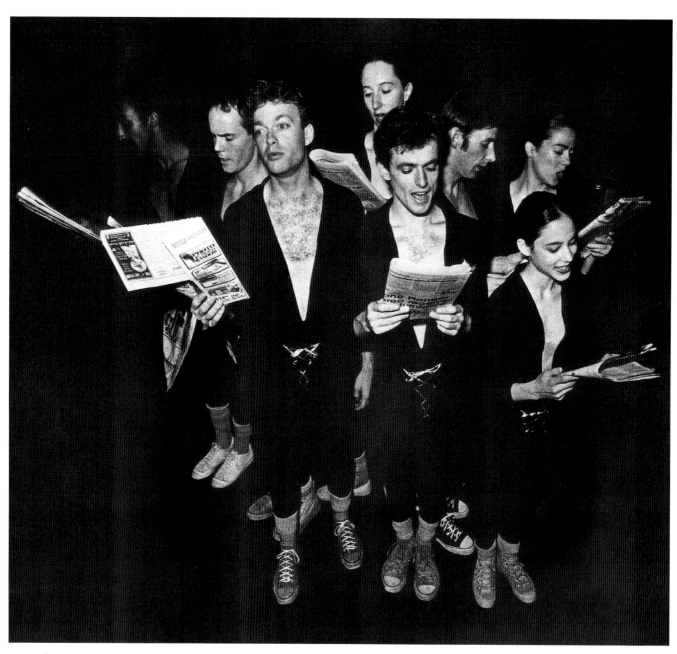

The Bridge, a complex blend of satire and barely repressed menace, was choreographed by Paula Ross for her Vancouver-based company in 1981. The piece was based, she said at the time, on her contrasting reactions to the growth of Vancouver. (Tamio Wakayama photograph)

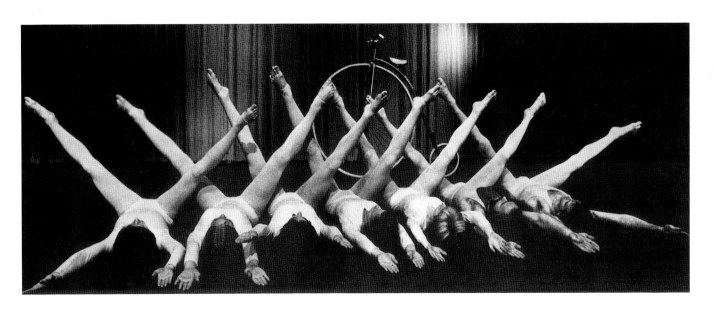

Dance is this . . . and this . . . and this became a signature-work for Vancouver's Anna Wyman Dance Theatre in the 1970s. The piece, choreographed by Wyman, demonstrated parallels between human and mechanical movement, and between athletic performance and dance. (Courtesy Anna Wyman Dance Theatre)

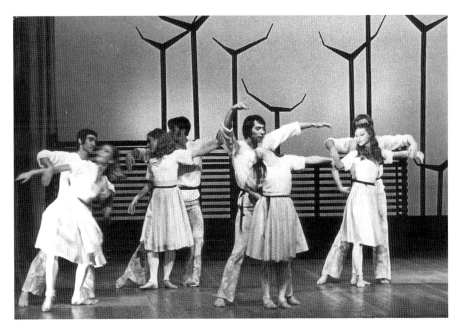

Norbert Vesak choreographed *Chichester Psalms,* to Leonard Bernstein's music, for his short-lived Western Dance Theatre in 1970. Dancers in couples (*left to right*): Ed Nichols and Teresa Bjornson, David Chase and Jane Erickson, Norbert Vesak and Gisa Cole, Tom McDevitt and Debbie Henry. (Dave Roels photograph)

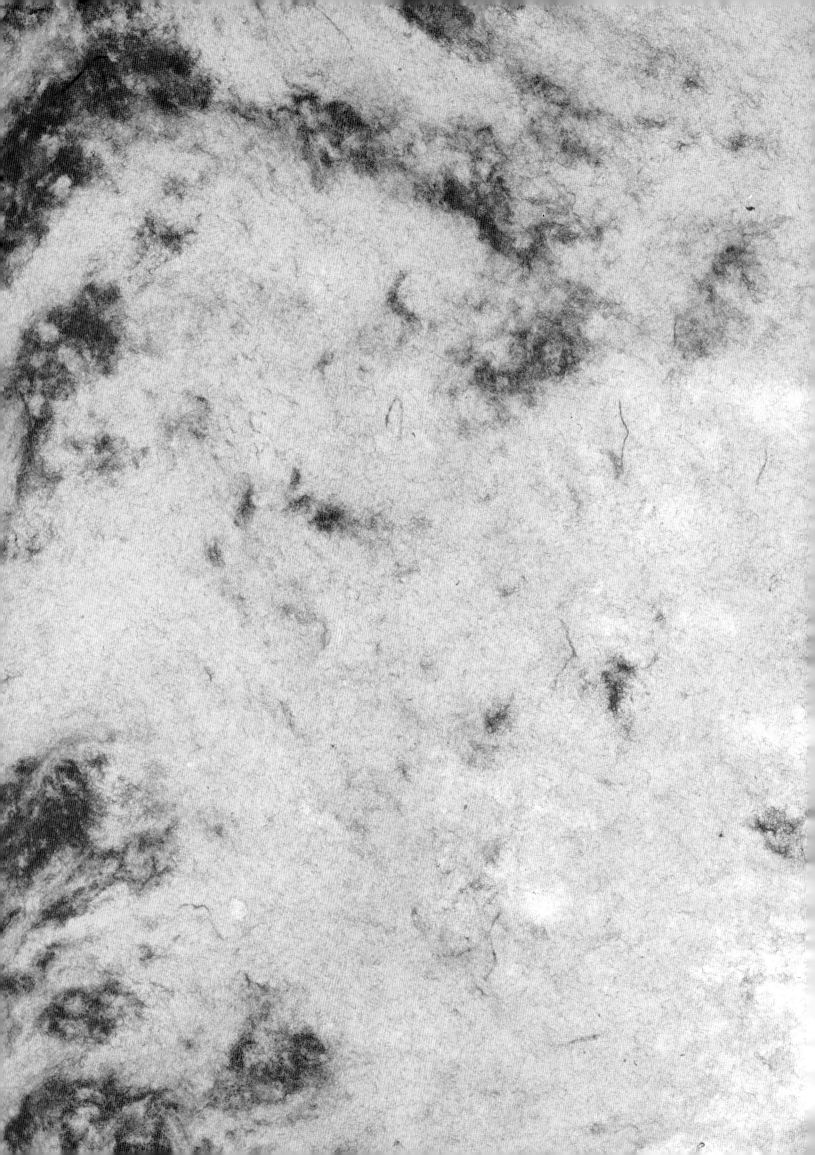

MODERN TIMES

Ballet

THE FLOWERING

In the late 1960s the body became (in the fashionable language of the time) the place where you found yourself, where you became centred; and the art form of the body attracted new chic. As the body became liberated, the imaginative response—the assertion of the human spirit—became bolder. The exuberance and freedom of the youth of the early sixties became common currency, and the corset of prejudice and prior definition into which art had been laced was slowly loosened.

For dance in Canada, the end of the 1960s and the beginnings of the 1970s were a golden age of optimism, experiment and expansion. Expo 67 and the centennial celebrations showed a surprised nation it had within itself the seeds of genuine exuberance and creative anarchy. And in the years that followed, the nation saw an efflorescence of new, vigorous, even challenging art. In a single season, 1966–67, the audience for ballet in Canada more than doubled—from 270,000 to 620,000.

Expo and the centennial also made the arts politically desirable—as image-enhancers abroad, and as tools to develop and define a distinctly Canadian culture at home—and as the political desirability of the arts grew, the purse-strings loosened. Funding for the Canada Council rose consistently; in 1972 the council, which had previously funded dance through the theatre office, established a separate dance section. In the same period, government make-work programmes for young people provided an unprecedented source of funding for experimental art.

A mood of excitement and readiness for change lay across the land.

———

In 1967, the National Ballet acquired two lavish new productions—a new *Nutcracker* by Franca and (its principal centennial project) a new *Swan Lake*, in an eccentric and controversial reworking by Erik Bruhn that discarded the traditional romantic-narrative approach in favour of psychodrama and symbolism.

The critics were split. In the *New York Times* Clive Barnes called the new *Swan Lake* "one of the great experimental versions of the ballet," and added that it confirmed the National Ballet as "one of the major North American companies." Nathan Cohen in the Toronto *Star* gave it a total thumbs-down. Choreographically, he said, the work was "primitive and querulous. Emotionally, it is soulless and barren. Dramatically, it is sketchy and muddled. In his effort to give it reality and logic, Bruhn has turned *Swan Lake* into a ballet for the birds."

Late the following year, Franca resigned abruptly. The company was in serious financial trouble (the accumulated deficit stood at $334,000—a third of the annual budget), most of the new Canadian works she had recently introduced had been poorly received, she was at loggerheads with her new business manager, and she was under pressure to hire a Frenchman, Roland Petit, to choreograph the new ballet the company had been asked to produce for the gala opening of the new National Arts Centre in Ottawa.

"I am used to criticism and have weathered much of it," she wrote to the board, "but I have always had enough support to carry on . . . I can't run the company's artistic affairs in an atmosphere of dissension, nor compromise my ideals beyond the point of honesty and self-respect." Within a month, a compromise was reached. Betty Oliphant was appointed associate artistic director to take some of the organizational burden from Franca's shoulders, and new management disciplines were introduced. But Franca's problems were far from over. The people at the National Arts Centre stuck to their guns and insisted that the National Ballet use Petit, rather than a Canadian choreographer, for their opening gala.

The opening was trumpeted as the highlight of the Canadian cultural year—and some considered it ironic that the very first performance seen at this handsome new showcase for Canada's artistic creativity should be a ballet choreographed by a Frenchman, to music by a Romanian Greek, conducted by a German American, with sets by a Hungarian . . . not one of them a resident of Canada.

The ballet itself, *Kraanerg*, was a flop. It lasted less than a dozen performances, was pulled out briefly three years later for the company's first visit to London, and after that was never seen again.

———

In Winnipeg, on the other hand, this was a period of unprecedented triumph. The company acquired work from four internationally famed choreographers (including new commissions from Eliot Feld and John Butler), and at their joint premiere performance in the fall of 1969, Clive Barnes in the *New York Times* had coined a set of phrases that were to characterize the RWB's image for years— "some companies," he wrote, "have a style; the Royal Winnipeggers have a manner. There is a buoyancy to the company, a kind of prairie freshness, warm and friendly and informal." Riding the crest of the wave, the bouncy Winnipeggers took two medals at the Paris International Festival and then went on to more successes in Leningrad and Moscow.

The Winnipeg company was the first to allow itself to be carried away on the tide of the sixties populism that was sweeping into every corner of Western culture. And Brian Macdonald provided works that precisely defined both style and era—an era in which caring had already begun to go commercial.

Marketing dance like cornflakes for the youth market, the RWB toured Canada in the fall of 1970 with what it called "one of the grooviest visual and sound treats to happen in Canadian theatre." It was an all-Macdonald bill that included *The Shining People of Leonard Cohen* (an unsensationally erotic response to the sentimental romanticism of the poetry that had captured the imagination of the hippie generation); *Ballet High* (a 90-minute set for the rock band Lighthouse, accompanied by the dancers of the RWB), and *Five Over Thirteen* (a message piece about the need for individual expression in a conformist society).

———

In Montreal, meanwhile, Les Grands Ballets used Expo year to strengthen its artistic position with a remounting of Fernand Nault's setting of Carl Orff's *Carmina*

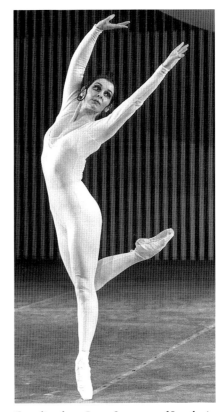

Canadian-born Lynn Seymour, of London's Royal Ballet, danced as guest artist in Roland Petit's Kraanerg *for the National Ballet of Canada at the opening of the National Arts Centre in Ottawa in 1969. She was partnered by Georges Piletta of the Paris Opera Ballet. (Ken Bell photograph)*

Burana, and a new production by Anton Dolin of *Giselle*, with Alicia Alonso, the Cuban-American ballerina, making her first North American appearance in seven years in the title role. Richard Buckle, of London's *Sunday Times*, fell in love with *Carmina Burana*—it should be in the repertoire of the Royal Ballet, he said—and Sydney Johnson, in the Montreal *Star*, called it "not only a theatrical achievement remarkable for Canada, but . . . probably quite unique on this continent." Nathan Cohen was respectful to Alonso's *Giselle* but he was scathing about the company. He saw, he said, "no evidence of the emergence of a point of view, of some real choreographic imagination, or of a company with any sense of cohesion and identity. Mostly, one gets a continuing impression of activity for its own sake."

But if the RWB threw itself willingly at the feet of the pop-culture generation that was emerging from the sixties, Les Grands Ballets stumbled over it almost by accident.

Their vehicle was *Tommy*, The Who's rock opera about a deaf-mute who becomes a pinball wonder, founds a new religion, and is turned against by his followers—the Christ parable described in the vivid musical terms of the sixties. No one expected a hit. Nault's setting of the music was scheduled for only four performances—"it was certainly not a conscious attempt to climb on the youth bandwagon," he said later. But it sold out, was remounted two months later, and, heavily toured, became financial salvation for the company.

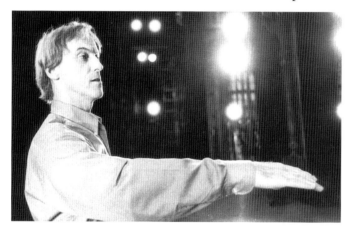

Uriel Luft, then manager of Les Grands, subsequently identified it as the start of the popular dance movement in Quebec. But dancer Vincent Warren saw it as the company's lowest artistic ebb. "The company went downhill, in terms of morale and technique, at the same time as it went up in terms of finance."

The choreography of Fernand Nault, an intensely religious person, has often carried strong spiritual overtones. Here he rehearses his Cérémonie, *a 1972 work that examined the theme of mystical love in a modern, physical world—"a gradual progression," he said, "from dark to light, from carnal to spiritual." (Courtesy Les Grands Ballets Canadiens)*

———

By now, all three ballet troupes were defining themselves by the choreographic company they kept. While the RWB and Les Grands wooed and wowed the world with schlock rock, the National stayed aloof from the trends of the time, devoting its energies to new Canadian choreography (three new works by untried choreographers on a single programme in 1971—a disaster) and the acquisition of a classic that was to become its signature-piece, Rudolf Nureyev's version of *The Sleeping Beauty*.

The Nureyev project began when New York impresario Sol Hurok invited the company to undertake a tour of the U.S. with the Soviet star in the fall of 1972. Franca did not like the idea of her company being used as a vehicle for Nureyev, with the star taking most of the male lead dancing, but the benefits (financial security, the addition of a major classic to the repertoire, and prolonged on-stage exposure for the dancers) outweighed her doubts, and the deal went ahead.

Almost immediately, costs started to escalate alarmingly. Designer Nicholas Georgiadis insisted on using only the finest materials for costumes; the sets included custom-built chandeliers and hunting coaches; Nureyev's casting demanded a specially enlarged company of 60 and a small army of supernumeraries.

What began as a ballet budgeted at $250,000 finally came in at well over $400,000—and while that expense was eventually repaid many times over at the *Sleeping Beauty* box office, Franca never overcame her basic reservations about both the ballet and its creator. She found the production tasteless and the choreography "stinking." And she didn't like the effect Nureyev had on the dancers. "If screaming and shouting and swearing is good, then he was good, but . . . there's a difference between temper and temperament. He considers he was of great artistic assistance to the company; in my opinion, he was not."

Not everyone agreed. Veronica Tennant remembered Nureyev warmly—"He said we were naive, and called us provincial, in a very loving way, but he helped everybody."

Franca believes Nureyev "ruined" Karen Kain by forcing her into the epic Beauty role too early, but Kain has a different view. "He taught me so much about dancing with, and to, a partner," she once told Tobi Tobias in *DanceMagazine*. "He showed me how essential it is really to relate, so that the audience can pick up that emotional excitement."

THE BLIGHT BENEATH THE BLOOM

The dancers of the National Ballet of Canada—said *DanceMagazine*'s Olga Maynard, in an article in the company's souvenir books of the early 1970s—"have a promise like springtime's, quick and urgent. To see them dance is to be witness to that charming phenomenon, when the dew is on the rose."

Invisible beneath the bloom, however, was the blight—not only in the National Ballet, but throughout the three principal professional companies in Canada. The nation's mood had changed. The excitement that had characterized the late 1960s had abated; now, all three companies were to undergo major crises and changes of direction and personnel.

Franca's departure from the National Ballet was a messy one. Her ongoing battle over artistic direction with manager Wallace Russell had led to Russell's abrupt resignation in 1972 and his replacement, on a temporary basis, by David Haber, a former Ruth Sorel dancer who had risen through a career in stage management, touring production and concert presentation to the post of programme director of the National Arts Centre.

Franca and Haber got on so well that by the end of 1972 he had been appointed co-artistic director, and eighteen months later Franca stepped aside to become company coach, clearing the way for Haber to become sole artistic director. The move was widely condemned in the dance community, where Haber's lack of experience as either a choreographer or dancer was seen as a distinct disadvantage. Betty Oliphant resigned as associate artistic director, declaring she didn't believe Haber had the qualifications to make artistic decisions alone—an action that infuriated her former friend, Franca. And in the spring of 1975, Haber himself was asked to resign.

Franca, backed into a corner by her loyalty to Haber, felt obliged to resign as

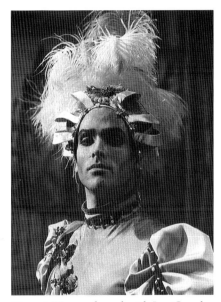

Vincent Warren danced with Les Grands Ballets Canadiens from 1961 to 1979. He is shown here in costume for Quatrième concert royale, *a work to music of Couperin in the style of Louis XIV, choreographed by Ludmilla Chiriaeff in 1961. (Courtesy Les Grands Ballets Canadiens)*

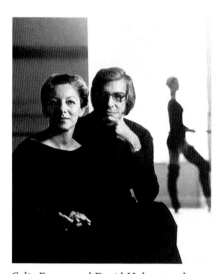

Celia Franca and David Haber together as co-artistic directors of the National Ballet of Canada in 1973. Haber was asked to resign in 1975 after the board refused to agree to his plans to mount a new production of Michel Fokine's 1914 work for Diaghilev, Le Coq d'or. (Anthony Crickmay photograph)

well, and while she stayed on as acting artistic director to help the company over the interim period while the board sought a permanent replacement, she confided, years later, that she always retained a sense of incompletion about her years with the company. She did return to take part in the company's twenty-fifth anniversary celebrations, in 1976, but reluctantly; under the façade of celebration she was (in her own words) "still a little heartbroken."

By the fall of 1975, a pall of gloom hung over the National Ballet of Canada. After the strong financial recovery of the Nureyev season of 1972–73, performances and attendances had slumped steadily, and the Haber-Franca debacle had badly sapped morale.

Into this morass parachuted Alexander Grant, a 30-year veteran of the Royal Ballet and since 1971 director of Ballet for All, a small touring offshoot of the company. Chosen from a multinational list of 63 candidates, Grant was at first by no means sure he wanted the job, and he went for advice to Ninette de Valois, the woman who had been so instrumental in sending Franca to Canada. He caught her in the crush bar at the Royal Opera House. "Madam, the National Ballet . . ." he began. Before he could get any further, she said: "Take it."

His arrival in Toronto as artistic director in July 1976 was seen as the start of a new phase of growth for the company. Like Franca, he brought with him a valuable dowry. Hers was Tudor, his was Ashton; between 1976 and 1981 five Ashton works were introduced, along with a range of other modern pieces from Europe and, in 1981, one of the company's most handsome successes, Peter Schaufuss's staging of the full-length Bournonville classic, *Napoli*.

At the same time, there was growing discontent within the company over the lack of opportunity for rising talent. A season contains only a limited number of nights, and a limited number of parts a night. Grant inherited a team headed by five ballerinas (including Karen Kain, whose international successes with Frank Augustyn in the mid-1970s had swung much of the focus her way); between them and the regular guests stars, there often wasn't much room left for the improving newcomers.

Grant had hoped from the start to be able to ease this pressure by the creation of a touring chamber ensemble. Financial constraints thwarted those hopes, but in 1979 a group of dancers from the company—Kain and Augustyn among them—set up a small touring company of their own. Ballet Revue was intended, said Ann Ditchburn, to let dancers show audiences aspects of their personalities that might not be seen in the standard National Ballet repertoire. Its programming mixed virtuoso classical showpieces with more modern and adventurous work, much of it by Ditchburn herself, and it toured Canada that spring.

However, plans to make its appearance a regular event never came to fruition—and the creative and artistic frustration that caused its creation was to get worse.

Alexander Grant was asked for his resignation by the National Ballet board in June 1982, a year before his contract was due to expire.

The company had reached a serious internal crisis. Two of its most promising choreographers, Ann Ditchburn and James Kudelka, had quit, claiming they needed more congenial working surroundings, and Kain and Augustyn had been highly critical of the lack of challenge in the repertoire. There were complaints that Grant, a generous and gentle man, lacked the necessary authority to rule a major arts organization. Audiences were down.

Grant called the request for his resignation a stab in the back, and remained bitter for years. He thought the dancers might have expected too much in the way of personal direction, rather than forging their own artistic development. And he stood proudly by his record: he had increased opportunities for young choreographers, he had diversified the repertoire by increasing the number of mixed programmes, he had brought in *Napoli* (expensive, but a significant artistic success) and he had acquired John Cranko's *Onegin* (which became, after Grant's departure, one of the pillars of the company repertoire).

But it was clearly not enough to satisfy the board, and by the summer of 1983 Grant had gone.

———

In Winnipeg, meanwhile, the RWB was having an identity crisis of its own. According to dancers who were there at the time, Macdonald had become increasingly demanding and difficult to work with.

He was also increasingly ambitious, directing in turn the Royal Swedish Ballet, the Harkness Ballet in New York, and the Batsheva company in Israel. Now he tried to enlist Winnipeg support in his bid to establish a new ballet company at the National Arts Centre in Ottawa. The Winnipeg board refused to help him, and according to one former board member, "he went off in a huff." He never made another ballet for the company.

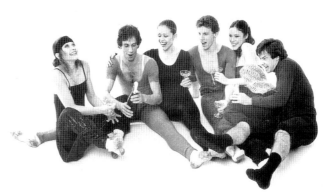

The six members of the short-lived Ballet Revue celebrate its 1979 launching. Left to right: *Ann Ditchburn, Tomas Schramek, Cynthia Lucas, David Roxander, Karen Kain and Frank Augustyn. (David Street photograph)*

His Ottawa company, Festival Ballet of Canada, made its debut in the summer of 1973, with his own new Romeo and Juliet ballet, *Star Cross'd*, but the National Arts Centre board decided to drop it after only a season.

The failure did nothing to deter Macdonald from his aim to become head of a company in Canada, and soon he got Les Grands Ballets Canadiens.

———

The albatross of *Tommy* hung about Les Grands Ballets throughout the early 1970s. It remained their best money-maker, but the critics hated it and the dancers were tired of it. Worst of all, it was becoming the company's signature-piece. They had searched long and hard for a distinctive identity. Was that search to end in *Tommy*?

In the summer of 1973, the company was broke, and *Tommy* was hauled out again. Ludmilla Chiriaeff took her case to the premier, Robert Bourassa. Even with *Tommy* selling out nightly, she said, they couldn't break even. Without more support, they might as well close down. Eventually, the government came through, but the struggle had been a frustrating and exhausting one, and in May 1974, Chiriaeff, her husband and company manager Uriel Luft, associate director Fernand Nault and executive secretary Guy Lamarre resigned in a body.

Macdonald was waiting. Part of the reason he hadn't been involved with Les Grands far earlier—it was his hometown company, after all—lay in wounded artistic pride. When he had launched Montreal Theatre Ballet more than a decade previously, he had been involved in a battle with Chiriaeff over dancers—"They had to make a choice," according to one senior member of the company, "and they chose Madame." But by the early 1970s the rift had healed, and Macdonald had not only made a couple of ballets for the company but also borrowed some of its dancers, with Chiriaeff's full encouragement, for the abortive Ottawa endeavour.

In 1974 he took over as artistic director, trailing a reputation as a demanding disciplinarian. Dancers who did not match his requirements found their contracts were not renewed. Some found conditions intolerable and simply quit. But he also brought new talents to the surface—among them Sylvie Kinal-Chevalier, who won a silver medal at the Varna contest in 1976, when she was 16, and less than a year later was thrust into the limelight as a last-minute stand-in for an injured Annette av Paul in a production of *Roméo et Juliette* (a remake of *Star Cross'd*).

As far as repertoire was concerned, said Macdonald, he would follow "guidelines set over a period of years in creating new things with a frankly Canadian ambience, while not excluding the classics." He concentrated on the creative side and left many other aspects of direction to his assistants, Linda Stearns and Daniel Jackson. The "frankly Canadian ambience" ranged from his own *Tam Ti Delam* (based on a collection of songs by Quebec chansonnier Gilles Vigneault) to an evening-long tribute to the memory of composer and TV producer Pierre Mercure.

As the repertoire improved, however, the atmosphere within the company grew steadily worse. Finally, during a tour of Latin America in 1977, the dancers organized a petition for Macdonald's removal, and that fall Macdonald's status changed from artistic director to resident choreographer. He was succeeded by a committee made up of Colin McIntyre, who had been general manager since 1975, Stearns and Jackson. With the pressures of directing removed and the animosity of the dancers lessened, Macdonald now proceeded to create some of his finest work—particularly *Double Quartet*, set to Schubert's *String Quartet in C Minor*, and R. Murray Schafer's *String Quartet No. 1*.

REBOUND: Changes in Direction

As their individual identities began to assume a greater clarity, all three of the country's principal ballet companies experienced inproving fortunes from the 1970s on.

In Winnipeg, Arnold Spohr's developing genius for spotting new choreographic talent, often years ahead of other companies, came into full play. Brian Macdonald had been his first discovery; now came Norbert Vesak and John Neumeier, two choreographers who would be as effective as Macdonald (though in radically different ways) in casting recognizable, salable images for the company.

Betty Farrally had seen the work of Vesak in Vancouver; she suggested that Spohr bring him to the Banff summer school to do some choreography. Spohr was impressed by what he saw, and when the Manitoba Indian Brotherhood approached the company in 1970 with the idea of producing a ballet to mark the centenary of the signing of certain local treaties, he asked Vesak to make a dance version of *The Ecstasy of Rita Joe*, George Ryga's sad and eloquent play about the death of an Indian girl in the big city. *Rita Joe* was introduced at the National Arts Centre in July 1971. Its social-issues theme and striking theatricality made it one of the biggest money-spinners in RWB history.

Not long after that, Vesak resettled in the United States, where he established a career as an opera choreographer and director. His subsequent connections with Canada were infrequent—though the *Belong* pas de deux from his second commission for the RWB, *What to Do Till the Messiah Comes*, became one of the company's most popular showpieces. Danced by Evelyn Hart and David Peregrine on their medal-winning trips to Varna and Osaka in 1980, *Belong* also took the gold medal for choreography at both events, a feat no choreographer had ever achieved before. Cables of congratulation reached Vesak from both Prime Minister Pierre Trudeau and the National Endowment for the Arts in Washington—both claiming him as a native son.

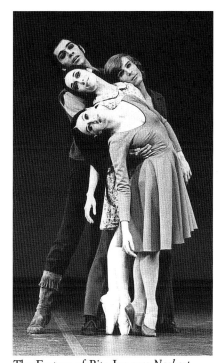

The Ecstasy of Rita Joe was Norbert Vesak's first commission for the Royal Winnipeg Ballet, in 1971. Based on the tragic play by George Ryga about the misadventures of an Indian girl who leaves the reserve for the bright lights of the city, it won the hearts of audiences around the world. (Colette Masson photograph)

Introduced on the same bill as *The Ecstasy of Rita Joe* was *Rondo*, by John Neumeier, later acknowledged as one of the most important choreographers to emerge in Europe in two decades. But at the time Spohr grabbed him (acting on a tip from Olga Maynard of *DanceMagazine*), he was virtually unknown in North America, and over a three-year period the RWB was able to acquire from him not only another consistent money-maker (his version of *Nutcracker*, a smiling love-poem to nineteenth-century ballet) but also a series of works that were to give the company a new air of artistic substance, dimension and durability.

And while Spohr was never to abandon the audience that wanted entertainment and drama (in 1973, for instance, he introduced Agnes de Mille's 1942 classic, *Rodeo*—for years something of a populist signature-piece for the company), he now began to move toward a more modernist look.

Yet another Spohr discovery, spotted in a dusty theatre in Buenos Aires during the company's Latin American tour in 1974, was Oscar Araiz—another choreographer well known on his home territory but virtually unknown in North America. In three years Araiz gave the RWB eight ballets—among them his brutalist setting of *Sacre du printemps* and his lush, romantic *Mahler IV: Eternity Is Now*. For a time, it was Araiz's work that defined most strongly this move toward dance that was, in Spohr's words, "of now." The RWB was growing up. But it didn't please everyone.

The risk-taking provoked a palace coup. As Gweneth Lloyd, Betty Farrally, David Yeddeau and Paddy Stone joined well-wishers from around the continent to share 40 pink birthday cakes and celebrate Spohr's achievements at the company's fortieth anniversary celebrations in 1978, a group of staff members and dancers opposed to the artistic thrust of the company made an unsuccessful bid to unseat Spohr. When the smoke cleared away, the company had lost 11 of its 26 dancers, and five key members of its artistic and administrative staff. Spohr referred to it laconically as "another cleaning-up time"—but it also gave him the impetus to refocus the company.

He switched his emphasis away from Araiz toward the hot young choreographers of Holland, with the importation of works by Rudi van Dantzig and Hans van Manen of the Dutch National Ballet. On the stage, the enforced infusion of fresh dancing talent, much of it from David Moroni's professional division of the company school, gave the RWB a noticeably vivacious look. "There was a time," Spohr said, "when I would have been afraid of replacing so many dancers. But the strength of the company now is the school."

It was the school, after all, that had produced the company's first real classical ballerina, Evelyn Hart, and it was Hart—and her successes in international competition—that gave Spohr the opportunity to move the company in the direction of the full-length classics, as a solid backbone for the familiar diversity of repertoire. He added Rudi van Dantzig's full-evening version of *Romeo and Juliet* in 1981, *Giselle* in 1982, and *Swan Lake* in 1984. All three became great personal successes for Hart.

The move toward the major classics was a radical modification of the RWB image, and the financial implications caused alarm in Ottawa. With a membership of 26 dancers, the company wasn't built to handle the full-lengths effectively (though Spohr solved that by using students from the professional programme). And another Canadian company had already laid firm claim to the classics.

Spohr was undisturbed. Maybe it did seem like an unexpected departure for his company. But he had not built the RWB into one of the greatest success stories in the contemporary Canadian arts by following the approved route. This was the culmination of a dream he had nursed for more than a quarter of a century. Finally, he said, he was seeing his hopes for the company realized.

————

Les Grands Ballets was also growing up. Searching for the company's elusive identity, the committee that took control after Macdonald introduced a broad sampling of the international twentieth-century repertoire—John Butler, Paul Taylor, Lar Lubovitch, José Limón, even Tudor's *Jardin aux lilas*.

James Kudelka's decision to leave the National Ballet of Canada and become a principal dancer with Les Grands Ballets Canadiens in 1981 had proven a stroke of good fortune for the Montreal company. Although Kudelka initially retained his connections as a choreographer with the National Ballet, he made for Les Grands Ballets a body of work that reinforced his growing international reputation as what the *New York Times* called "one of the best young choreographers to turn up in ballet in recent years."

When the company returned to New York in 1982, it impressed Anna Kisselgoff of the *New York Times* with the percentage of recent works it was prepared to show. Les Grands Ballets, she said, was "one of the few companies seen hereabouts that does not seem to be suffering from hardening of the toe-shoes. That is, it seems to be willing to court risk as well as success."

Despite its New York acclaim, the company itself had fluctuating fortunes, and in 1985 took a major change of artistic direction with the replacement of the triumvirate of Linda Stearns, Colin McIntyre and Daniel Jackson by a pair of co-artistic directors, Stearns and Jeanne Renaud. McIntyre had in any case already left the company to put together an exhibition centred on the work of Diaghilev; Jackson joined modernist Paul-André Fortier to create Montréal Danse.

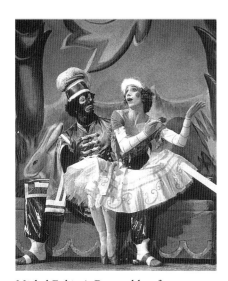

Michel Fokine's Petrouchka, *first presented by the Diaghilev Ballets Russes in Paris in 1911, was restaged for Les Grands Ballets Canadiens in the 1988–89 season by John Aulds. Shown here are Kevin Irving as the Blackamoor and Gioconda Barbuto as the Ballerina. (Michael Slobodian photograph)*

Renaud was brought in because of her close ties with the experimental dance community in Montreal. She talked at the time of developing a company that would explore the innovative edge while still maintaining its neoclassical strengths, and soon the company was mixing familiar fare like *Giselle* and George Balanchine's *Concerto Barocco* with new ventures by Kudelka (including a version of *Dracula* starring the solo modern dancer Margie Gillis), and modernist experimenters Edouard Lock of La La La Human Steps and Christopher House of Toronto Dance Theatre.

———

Erik Bruhn was artistic director of the National Ballet for barely three years before his death from cancer at the age of 57 in 1986. But in those years he transformed a precisely calibrated dancing machine into a fine-tuned expressive instrument.

Acknowledged as one of the finest *danseurs nobles* of the twentieth century, Bruhn was no stranger either to the National Ballet or to company directorship when he accepted the invitation to succeed Alexander Grant in 1983. He had spent four difficult years as head of the Royal Swedish Ballet in the late 1960s (one of his first acts was to invite Betty Oliphant to Stockholm to revamp the company school), and he could have been head of the Royal Danish Ballet (where he began) or American Ballet Theatre (where he was a principal for 20 years).

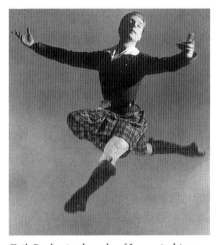

Erik Bruhn in the role of James in his own production of La Sylphide *for the National Ballet of Canada in 1964. He injured his knee and was replaced at the third performance by his friend Rudolf Nureyev. (Courtesy National Ballet of Canada)*

But he turned down all offers until Toronto. The National was different. The National was "family." He had partnered Celia Franca in London's Metropolitan Ballet in the 1940s, and from 1964, when Franca had invited him to set *La Sylphide*, he had been a frequent visitor to the company, as teacher, coach, producer and choreographer.

It was also a challenge. He inherited a company that had always hovered nervously on the far side of promise. What he did was liberate it from its bonds of anxiety (about important but essentially petty matters like technical respectability, correctness, getting things *right*) and let its dancers reach beyond technique, as he so memorably had in his own career, and find their expressiveness as invididual human artists.

With characteristic assertion, but with exquisite courtesy and understanding, he took a bewildered and demoralized artistic enterprise by the shoulders, gave it a series of firm shakes, and proceeded to infuse it with new purpose, new belief in itself, new vitality. He gave it the courage to assert the distinctive character it had always lacked, and forced it to be the best it could be. The best it could be was better than many had thought.

In terms of human feelings, the exercise was often costly. To make way for the new generation of performing talent that he saw emerging from the National Ballet School and the company's lower ranks, established dancers had to step aside. Not everyone was happy to do so.

But Bruhn insisted on his vision, displaying this new and rising generation in programming of fresh relevance and excitement.

The National Ballet was never merely a storehouse for the great classical treasures; Franca had consistently introduced new work, and so had Grant. But Bruhn embraced contemporaneity with a new boldness and vigour, acquiring works by Canadian modernists Danny Grossman and Robert Desrosiers, and coaxing a new ballet, *Alice*, from veteran U.S. choreographer Glen Tetley.

He also leaned on his friends for help. Mikhail Baryshnikov danced at a fund-raising gala in 1984—his first appearance in Toronto since his defection from the touring Kirov Ballet in the city a decade earlier. The same year, another Kirov defector, Natalia Makarova, staged a work for him, and yet another, Rudolf Nureyev, returned to the company to dance in his own *Sleeping Beauty*.

With his fresh demands for excellence in both programming and performance, Bruhn provided a key that unlocked the door leading from worthy performance to international achievement. At the time of his death, the company was just stepping over the threshold.

LESSER LIGHTS

Outside the three major ballet companies, Canada has had a variety of smaller professional ballet troupes, though ballet is such an expensive venture that the Canada Council for years has placed a limit on the size of small companies it is willing to support.

Longest-established of the small companies is the Alberta Ballet, founded by former Volkoff dancer Ruth Carse. Carse danced in the corps at Radio City Music Hall, spent a month in the first National Ballet company, and when injury ended her performing career in 1954, set up as a teacher and choreographer in Edmonton. Within a year she had launched a small, unpaid performing group, "to foster ballet in rural and urban Alberta," and was writing for advice to Gweneth Lloyd.

Lloyd wrote back sternly: "I think you should consider yourselves merely as people who can bring to the small communities a vision of something which otherwise they would have no conception of. It is possible to reach a degree of finish, especially with your knowledge and experience, which, combined with simple and not too erudite ideas, can give enormous pleasure to the rural communities."

So Carse equipped her little company with $1,000 worth of portable sets and lights and sent a show called Ballet Interlude on weekend tours through the small towns of Alberta—fantasy dances, story-ballets, comedy numbers, jazz routines and folk dances based on local ethnic traditions.

The company turned professional in 1966, but it was not until the arrival of Brydon Paige as artistic director ten years later that the Alberta Ballet made serious claims to international recognition. Paige's ambitions for the company were in the RWB league, and he built a safe, all-purpose repertoire that ranged from George Balanchine and Frederick Ashton to Norbert Vesak (whose *Grey Goose of Silence*, in 1981, was his first new work in Canada for almost a decade). Full-evening ballets were heavily featured, as was the work of Lambros Lambrou, resident choreographer for a decade. Paige quit as artistic director in 1987, at the height of the company's acclaim, to give himself more time to create. He was succeeded in 1988 by Iranian-American choreographer Ali Pourfarrokh, who began to move the company away from its strictly classical look toward a conservative modernity of repertoire and performance style.

The company's chief competition in Alberta has been the Calgary City Ballet, a professional company of ten dancers directed from 1981 to 1986 by Laszlo Tamasik. He was succeeded by Jean Leger.

Theatre Ballet of Canada, based in Ottawa, evolved from two earlier companies, Entre-Six and Ballet Ys. Entre-Six was founded in Montreal in 1975 by Lawrence Gradus, a former soloist with American Ballet Theatre who had moved to Les Grands Ballets Canadiens in 1969, and his wife, Jacqueline Lemieux, a teacher at Les Grands and a former Elizabeth Leese dancer. The company's approach was intimate and unpretentious, and Gradus took the Chalmers award for choreography in the company's first year. Lemieux managed the company virtually single-handedly, as well as launching and organizing Québec Eté Danse, an annual summer school. However, she died of cancer in 1979, at the age of 40; in the absences her illness had caused, Entre-Six had fallen into financial disaster, and within four months of her death the company folded.

Ballet Ys (the word means "of the times" in Gaelic) was founded in Toronto in 1971 and became a platform for new work in the crossover modern-ballet vein. However, by 1979 criticism of its direction was mounting, and artistic director Gloria Grant made it clear she wanted to relinquish control. Soon after, it was decided to improve the company's fund-raising potential by changing its name to Theatre Ballet of Canada. Talks to discuss a merger between Entre-Six and Ballet Ys were held, but broke off when the Ballet Ys people learned of the financial troubles of Entre-Six.

However, Gradus was hired as artistic director, and the new company made its debut at the National Arts Centre in Ottawa in February 1981. The program, dedicated to the memory of Jacqueline Lemieux, closed with the presentation of the Jacqueline Lemieux prize, subsequently an annual award from the Canada Council. The recipient was Robert Desrosiers, one of the first choreographers for Ballet Ys. Gradus was succeeded as artistic director in 1989 by Frank Augustyn.

Vancouver remained a resolutely modern-dance city until the mid-1980s, though there was never any shortage of attempts to establish professional ballet.

Performing groups regularly travelled to the ballet festivals—including Mara McBirney's Panto-Pacific Ballet in 1949 and the Heino Heiden Vancouver Ballet in 1954—and the Vancouver Ballet Society, established in 1946 to expand the experience of city dancers, regularly mounted major productions. Its 1961 showcase, inspired in part by the guest appearance the previous year of city daughter Lynn Seymour and her Royal Ballet partner Christopher Gable, was expected by some to lead to a permanent company. However, although the showcase productions of the 1960s featured performances by many dancers who were to become professionals, they never resulted in the formation of a company.

From time to time through the 1960s and 1970s other groups or individuals tried to launch Vancouver ballet troupes—among them a 1966 venture that teamed former Royal Ballet character dancer Franklin White with former Volkoff and Hollywood dancer Beth Lockhart; and Ballet Horizons, launched in 1971 by five former RWB dancers. They all foundered; spoiled by decades of exposure by local promoters to the cream of the world's ballet companies, Vancouver's dance

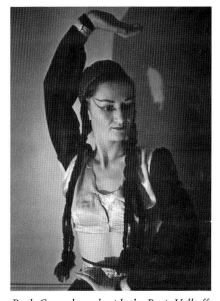

Ruth Carse danced with the Boris Volkoff company (she is shown here in costume for Prince Igor) *and in New York before settling in Edmonton in 1954 to launch the amateur group that became the Alberta Ballet. (Donnia V. Bax photograph, courtesy Ruth Carse)*

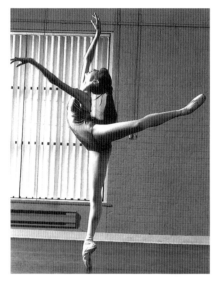

Chan Hon Goh trained with her father, Choo Chiat Goh, in Vancouver and danced with his company, the Goh Ballet. In 1987 she won a Prix de Lausanne at the Swiss city's annual contest for young dancers. She joined the National Ballet of Canada in 1988. (David Street photograph)

audiences were reluctant to support the struggles of indigenous professionalism.

Ballet B.C. was different. Launched in 1985 out of the ashes of yet another failed endeavour, Maria Lewis's Pacific Ballet Theatre, it set out to build itself a name. Principal artistic guidance initially came from Annette av Paul, former star with Les Grands Ballets Canadiens and wife of Brian Macdonald, but in 1987 she passed the reins to Reid Anderson, born in British Columbia and recently retired from a successful dancing career in Germany. Anderson, with access to the repertoire of Stuttgart's John Cranko, rapidly established for the company a "contemporary-ballet" identity, importing works from a variety of Europe's front-running ballet modernists, and persuading Natalia Makarova to be part of a gala that also featured a duo from the Kirov Ballet—the first time in 17 years the famous defector had appeared on the same stage as dancers from her home company. Anderson left Ballet B.C. to become artistic director of the National Ballet of Canada in 1989, and was replaced by Patricia Neary, a former Balanchine principal and director of ballet companies in Geneva and Milan.

Concurrently with the establishment of Ballet B.C., Singapore-born, Beijing-trained teacher Choo Chiat Goh launched in Vancouver the Goh Ballet, a company that attempted, with mixed success, to blend the Western and Chinese classical movement traditions. The company has twice toured the Orient.

Other small companies, often operating on an amateur basis, have appeared regularly across Canada. Many, predictably, have been in Ontario. Nesta Toumine tried several times to re-establish a company in Ottawa after the collapse of her venture with Yolande Leduc in 1949. Another prominent contributor to the growth of regional ballet was Diana Vorps, a Latvian teacher who arrived in Toronto in 1951 and later established the Toronto Regional Ballet. In 1977 Judith Davies established the Ottawa Dance Theatre as a touring ensemble presenting a range of dance styles. The Dance Company of Ontario, a small touring company created in 1979 by former National Ballet principal Lois Smith, with Earl Kraul as ballet master, collapsed in 1981 for lack of funds. Yugoslavian Marijan Bayer danced with the National Ballet for two years before launching the City Ballet of Toronto in 1973; in 1982 he moved to Halifax and renamed the troupe the Atlantic Ballet Company.

In Nova Scotia, the Halifax Ballet disintegrated after Jury Gotshalks and his wife Irene Apiné joined the National Ballet of Canada at its debut in 1951. Hilda Strombergs, principal dancer with the Halifax company, took a reconstituted ensemble, the Halifax Theatre Ballet, to the 1953 and 1954 festivals.

Montreal has also seen many small, sometimes transient companies, among them Pointépienu, founded in 1976 by Louise Latreille, a former dancer with Les Grands Ballets and with Belgium's Maurice Béjart, whose theatrical style has heavily influenced the company.

In Quebec City, serious dance activity has been sporadic. Georges Bérard's Ballets de Québec, launched in 1957, produced more than 20 works, but after its demise in 1964 there was nothing of note until the launching in 1976 of Dansepartout, founded by Chantal Belhumeur, another former dancer with Les Grands Ballets.

A quite dissociated dance phenomenon that emerged in the province of Quebec in the 1970s was the rise of jazz ballet.

It was stimulated primarily by the international success of Les Ballets Jazz, a company that synthesizes North American showdance and ballet into a new dance form. It originated with two women from European ballet backgrounds— Geneviève Salbaing, born in Paris and principal dancer with the Casablanca municipal ballet, and Budapest-born Eva von Gencsy, who danced with the Royal Winnipeg Ballet and Les Ballets Chiriaeff.

In Montreal, von Gencsy developed an enthusiastic coterie of followers, among them the Haiti-born Eddy Toussaint, and in 1972 she and Toussaint started Les Ballets Jazz, with Salbaing providing business guidance. Toussaint left within a year to develop his own company, and von Gencsy quit in 1979, leaving Salbaing in artistic control.

The company has toured widely, to extensive audience acclaim, though both Les Ballets Jazz and Ballet de Montréal Eddy Toussaint, founded in 1974, have come under consistent criticism for the lightweight character of their choreography. "I don't want to make my audiences think," Toussaint once said, though his highly theatrical style, slick, polished and sexy, gradually began to show in the early 1980s a deeper concern with pure ballet.

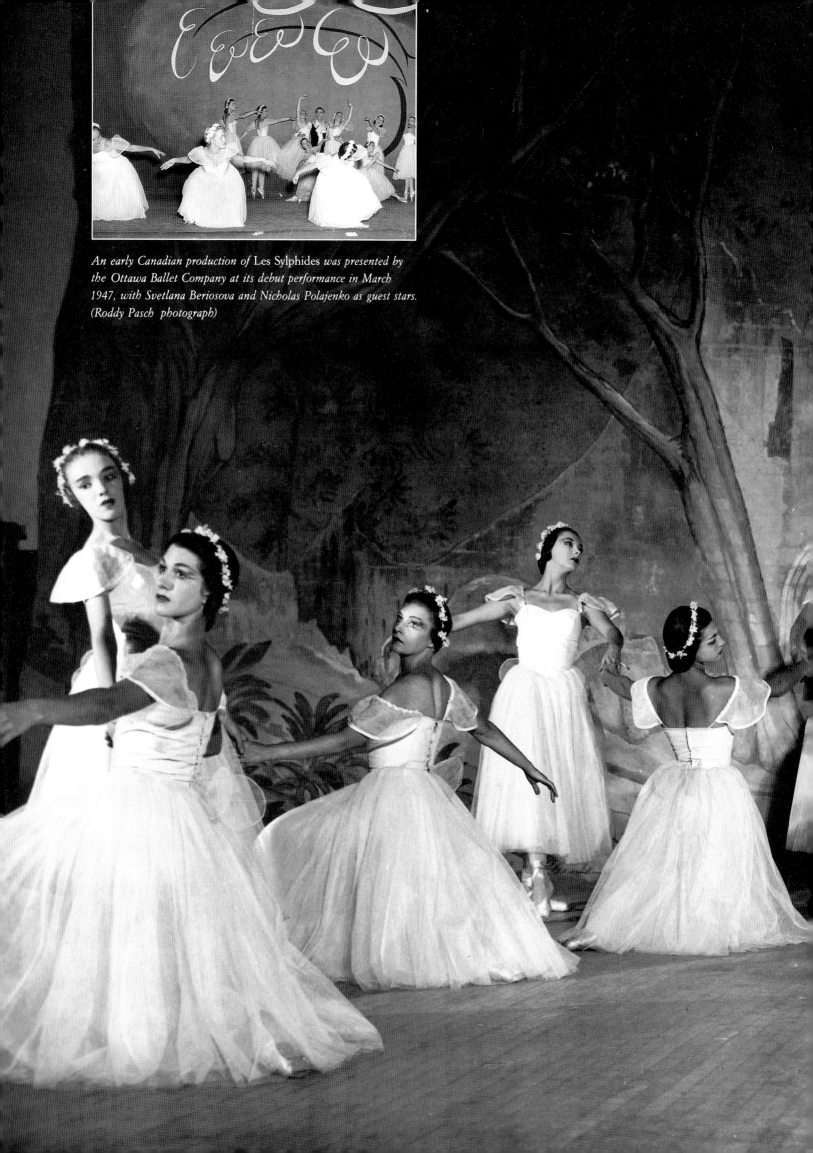

An early Canadian production of Les Sylphides *was presented by* the Ottawa Ballet Company *at its debut performance in March 1947, with Svetlana Beriosova and Nicholas Polajenko as guest stars.* (Roddy Pasch *photograph*)

Les Sylphides

Although many associate *Les Sylphides* with the Romantic period of the mid-nineteenth century, the ballet is actually a twentieth-century work. Michel Fokine presented it under the title *Chopiniana* at a 1908 charity performance in St. Petersburg. At that time it was a series of danced scenes, mostly in national costumes, to Glazunov's orchestration of Chopin piano pieces. Later, rechoreographed, recostumed and retitled, it entered the repertoire of the Diaghilev Ballets Russes in Europe. It is one of the loveliest and most poetic of all abstract *ballets blancs,* and a favourite of audiences everywhere. All three of Canada's principal ballet companies have versions in their repertoires.

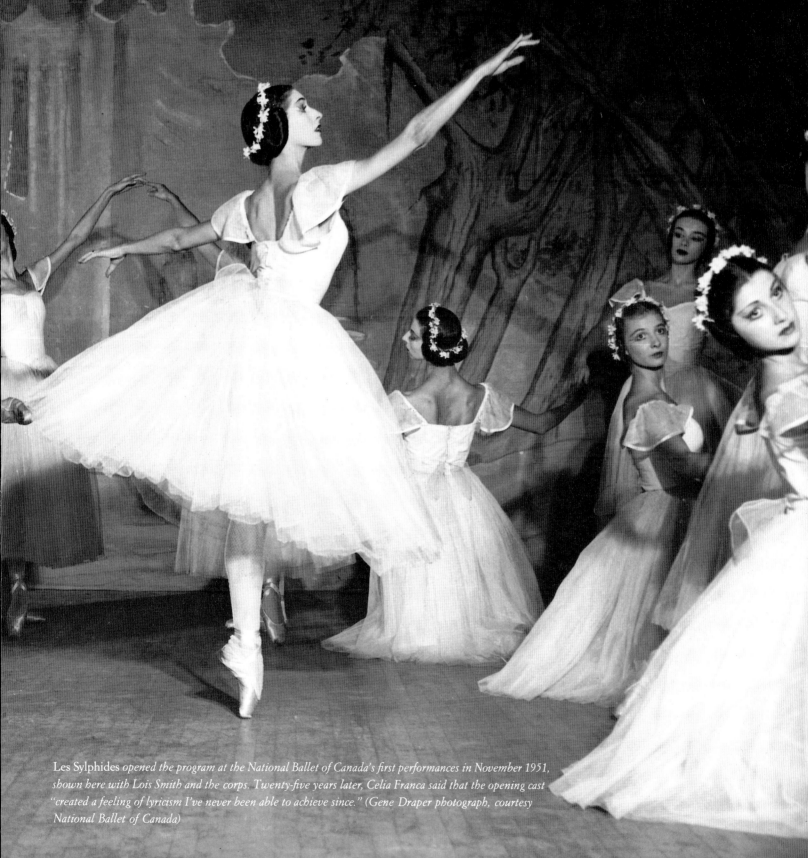

Les Sylphides opened the program at the National Ballet of Canada's first performances in November 1951, *shown here with Lois Smith and the corps. Twenty-five years later, Celia Franca said that the opening cast "created a feeling of lyricism I've never been able to achieve since." (Gene Draper photograph, courtesy National Ballet of Canada)*

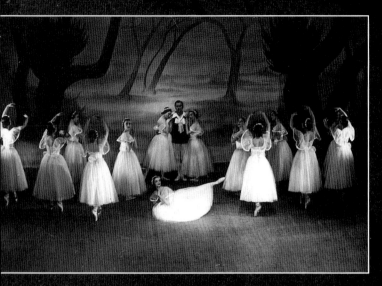

Alicia Markova, the English ballerina who co-founded the London Festival Ballet, danced in Les Sylphides *as guest artist with the Royal Winnipeg Ballet in 1953. She taught and coached the dancers and, disapproving of the corps costumes, paid to replace the top layers. (Courtesy Jean Stoneham Orr)*

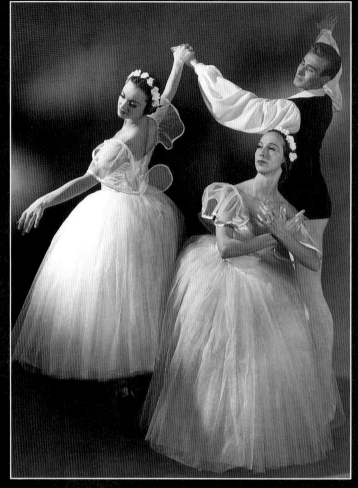

The Winnipeg Ballet mounted a production of Les Sylphides *in the fall of 1951. In this studio pose, Arnold Spohr is shown with Jean Stoneham (left) and Sheila Killough. (Phillips-Gutkin photograph)*

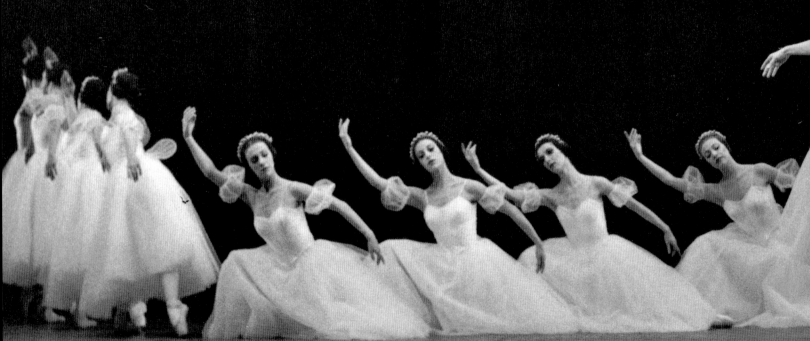

Les Grands Ballets Canadiens first performed Les Sylphides *in 1965. This photograph shows Louise Doré and the company women in a 1980 performance of Fernand Nault's staging. (Andrew Oxenham photograph)*

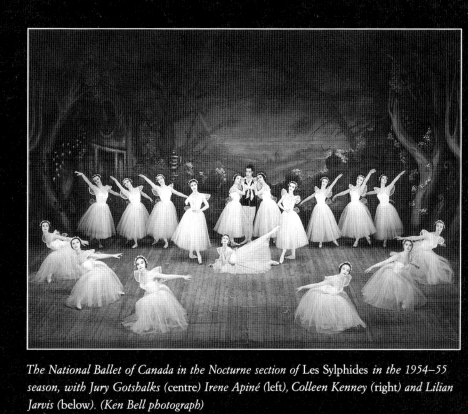

The National Ballet of Canada in the Nocturne section of Les Sylphides *in the 1954–55 season, with Jury Gotshalks* (centre) *Irene Apiné* (left), *Colleen Kenney* (right) *and Lilian Jarvis* (below). *(Ken Bell photograph)*

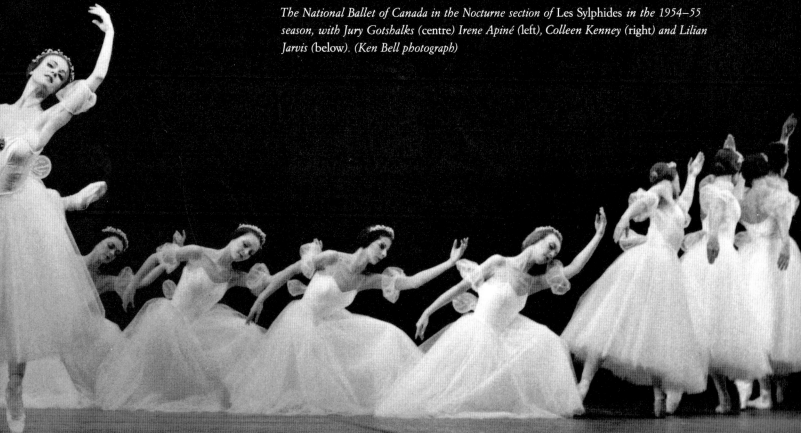

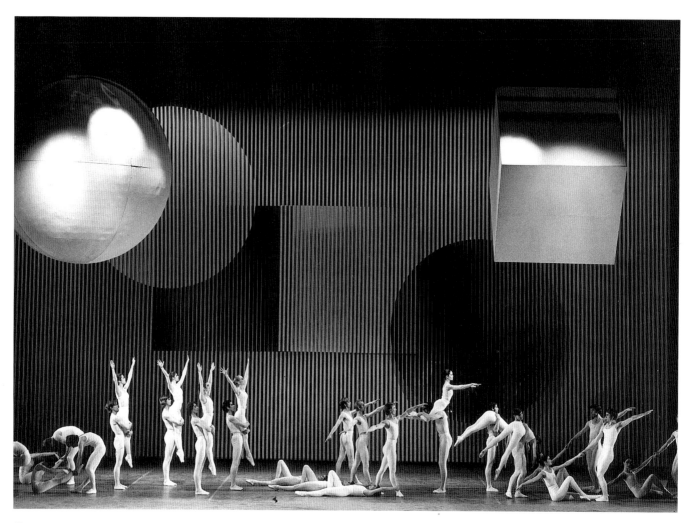

Kraanerg, commissioned from the French choreographer Roland Petit for performance by the National Ballet of Canada at the opening of the National Arts Centre in Ottawa in 1969, had mobile decors by Victor Vasarely and Yvaral, and music by Iannis Xenakis. (Ken Bell photograph)

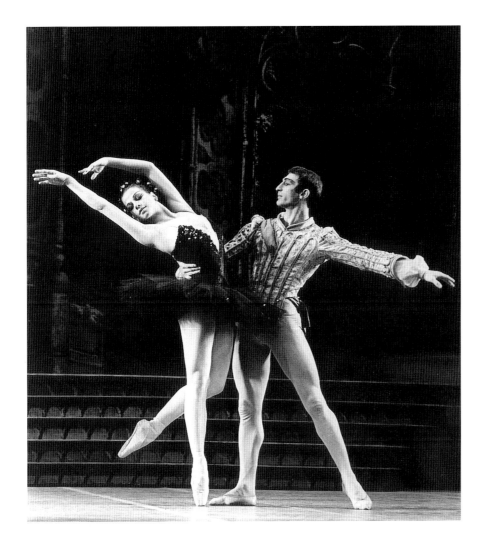

Martine van Hamel studied at the
National Ballet School and joined the
National Ballet of Canada as a soloist in
1963. She won the gold medal at the
Varna International Competition in 1966.
This photograph shows her opposite
Hazaros Surmeyan in the National Ballet's
Swan Lake in 1967. (Ken Bell photograph)

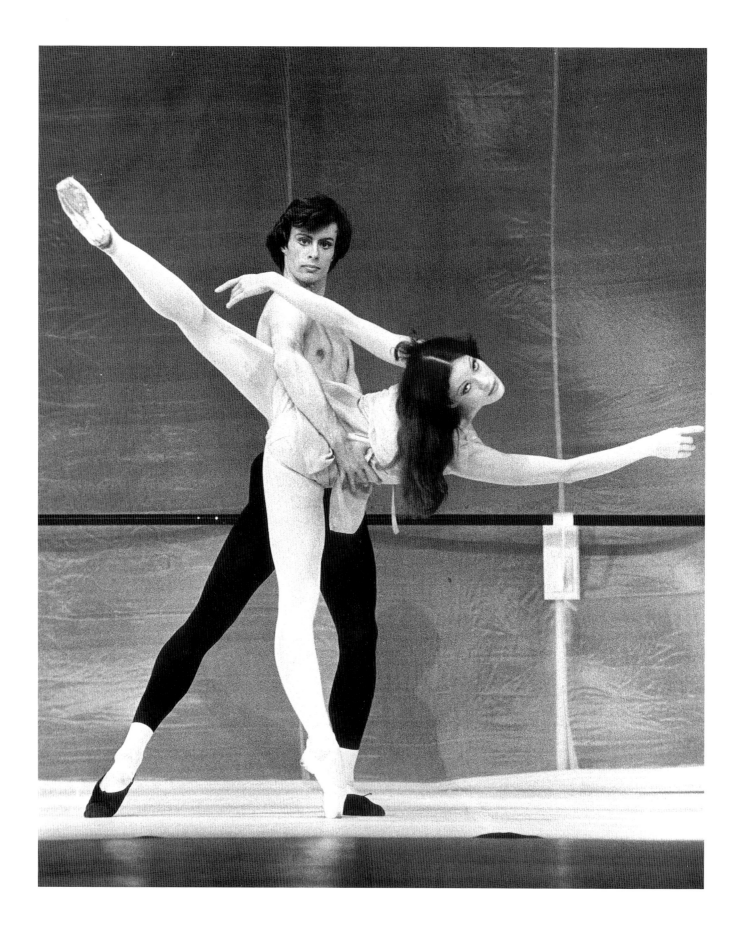

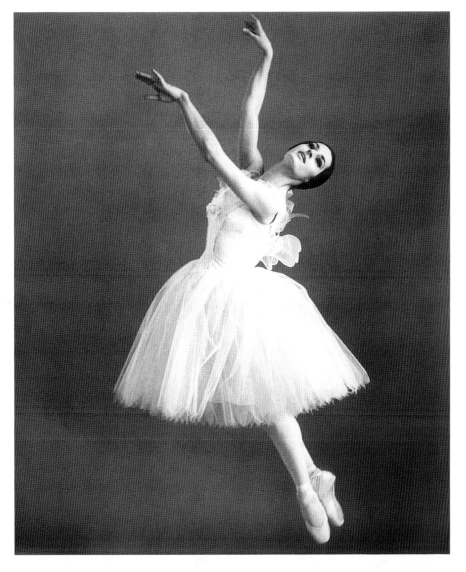

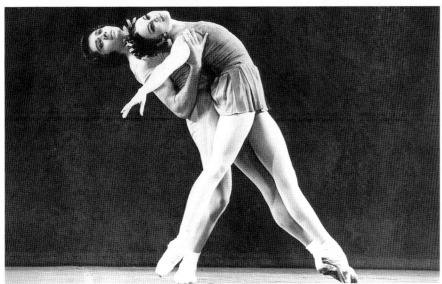

Facing page: Although Canada had famous dancing duos in the early years of ballet's development, Karen Kain and Frank Augustyn became the country's first international stars following their medal-winning success in Moscow in 1973. They are shown here in the National Ballet of Canada's production of Jerome Robbins's *Afternoon of a Faun,* in the 1976–77 season. (Barry Gray photograph)

In her 24-year career with the National Ballet of Canada, Veronica Tennant danced virtually every lead role in the repertoire. She appears here as Giselle in 1970. (Ken Bell photograph)

Vanessa Harwood entered the National Ballet of Canada in 1965, launching a career in dance that lasted more than 20 years. She appears here in the lead role in the company's production of Kenneth MacMillan's *Solitaire,* with Sergiu Stefanschi. (Courtesy National Ballet of Canada)

Mary Jago became a principal dancer with
the National Ballet of Canada in 1966,
after training and dancing in England. She
is shown here in John Neumeier's 1974
ballet for the company, *Don Juan.* Her
partner is principal dancer Sergiu
Stefanschi, Varna silver medallist in 1964,
who joined the company in 1971.
(Anthony Crickmay photograph)

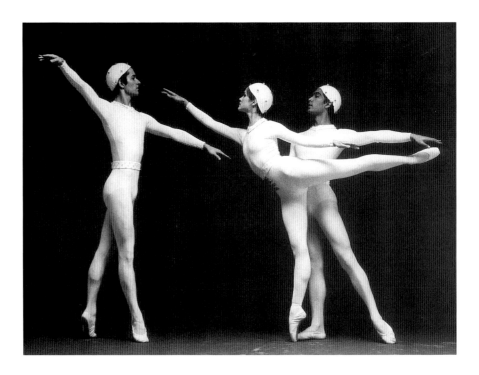

Frederick Ashton's *Monotones II,* to
Satie's *Trois Gnossienes,* is a popular short
work in many companies. It is shown here
in a performance from the National Ballet
of Canada's 1976–77 season, featuring
(*left to right*) James Kudelka, Nadia Potts
and Miguel Garcia. (Andrew Oxenham
photograph)

Facing page: Frank Augustyn joined the
National Ballet of Canada in 1970, and
three years later he and Karen Kain won
the prize for best pas de deux at the
Moscow International Ballet Competition.
He appears in this 1975 photo as the
Bluebird in the company's production of
The Sleeping Beauty, choreographed by
Rudolf Nureyev. (Anthony Crickmay
photograph)

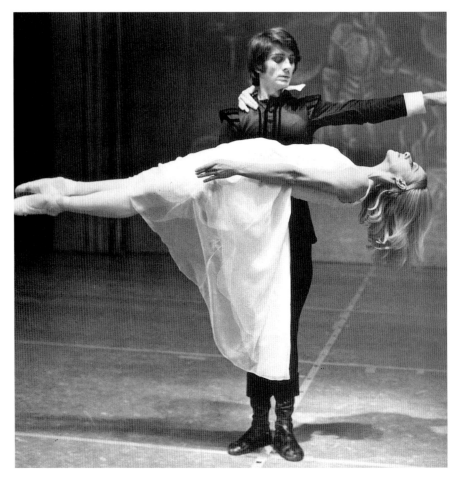

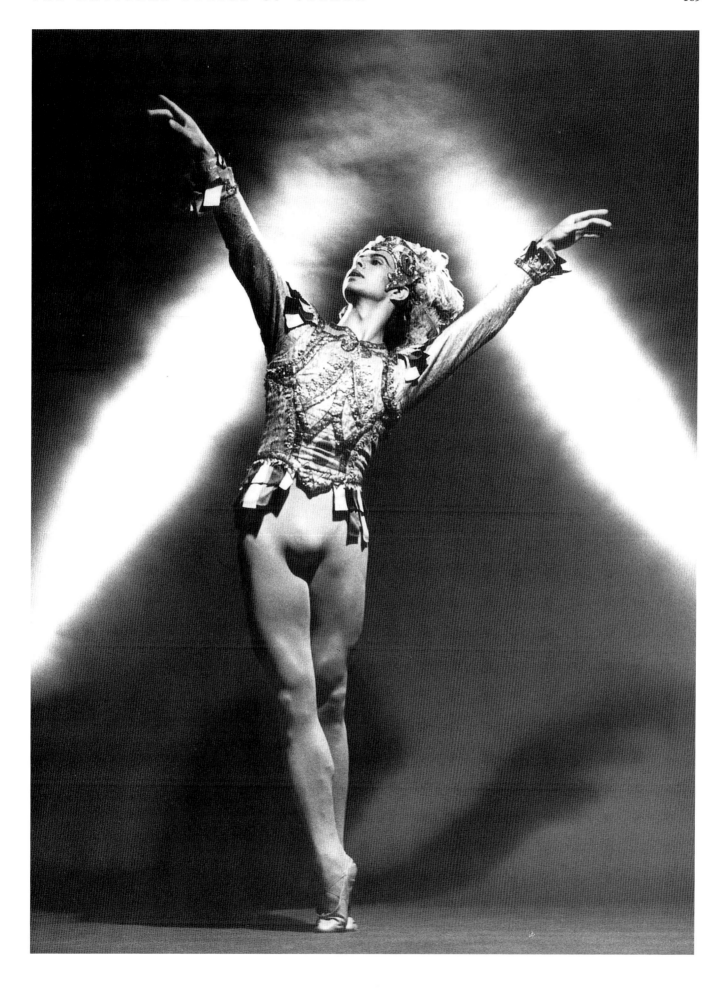

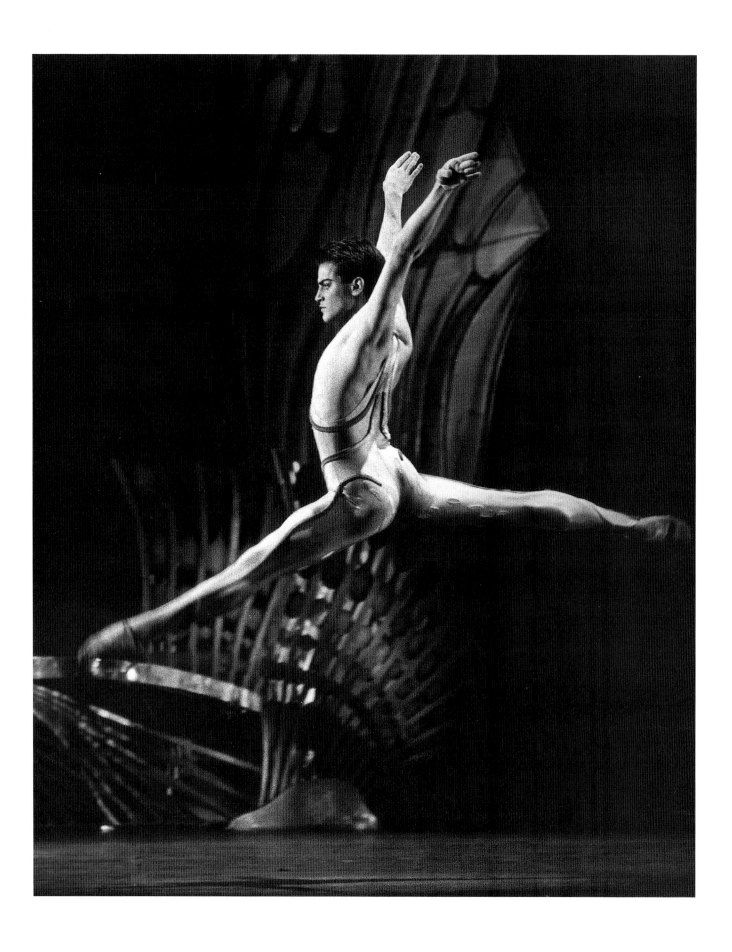

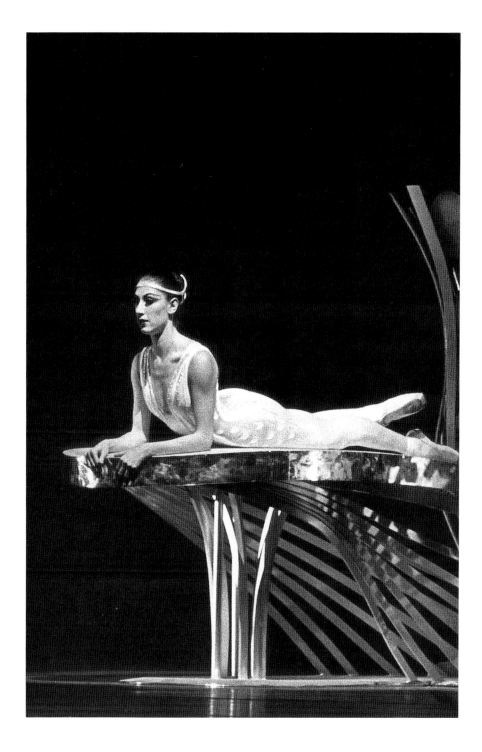

Facing page: Rex Harrington played Oedipus, the nemesis of *The Sphinx,* in Glen Tetley's 1982 work for the National Ballet of Canada. A graduate of the National Ballet School, Harrington was hailed as "an instant matinee idol" by *New York Times* dance critic Anna Kisselgoff. (Andrew Oxenham photograph)

Gizella Witkowsky played the title role in *The Sphinx,* made for the National Ballet of Canada by Glen Tetley in 1982. It was based on a Jean Cocteau play in which the Sphinx of Greek legend, wearying of her divinity, dreams of a man she can love as an equal. (Andrew Oxenham photograph)

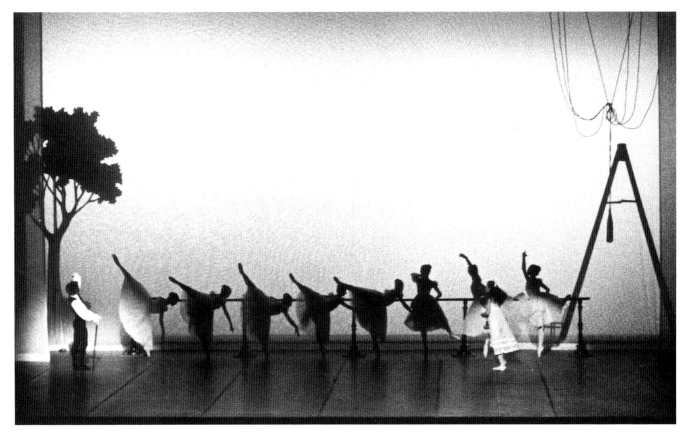

John Neumeier's version of *Nutcracker,* made for the Royal Winnipeg Ballet in 1972, dispensed with the traditional Christmas settings in favour of a balletic theme, with the young girl being transported not to a Land of Sweets but to a magical world of ballet. (Peter Garrick photograph)

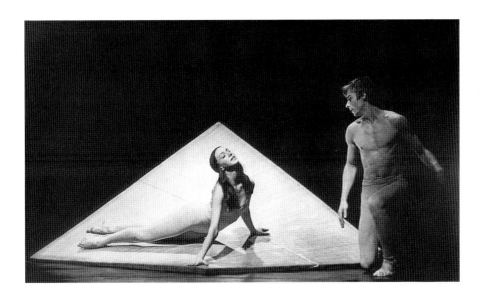

The Shining People of Leonard Cohen, made by Brian Macdonald for the Royal Winnipeg Ballet in 1970, was performed to a reading of Cohen's poems and an electronic sound montage by composer Harry Freedman. Sculptures by Ted Bieler provided the set. Shown are Madeleine Bouchard and Attila Ficzere. (Kopelow photograph, courtesy Royal Winnipeg Ballet)

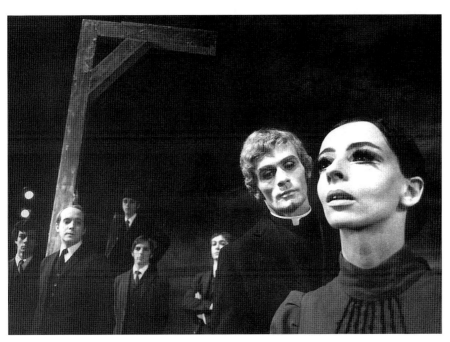

Agnes de Mille's *Fall River Legend,* based on the true story of the Lizzie Borden axe-murders, was made in 1948 and entered the Royal Winnipeg Ballet repertoire in 1969. It was one of five de Mille works either acquired or commissioned by the RWB. In this 1970 photograph, David Moroni plays the Pastor and Christine Hennessy is the Accused. (Martha Swope photograph)

Overleaf: The Rite of Spring by Oscar Araiz was acquired by the Royal Winnipeg Ballet in 1975. Danced in brief rehearsal costumes on a bare stage, it is a savage and erotic treatment of the Stravinsky music. Shown here: Sheri Cook as the Earth Spirit. (Peter Garrick photograph)

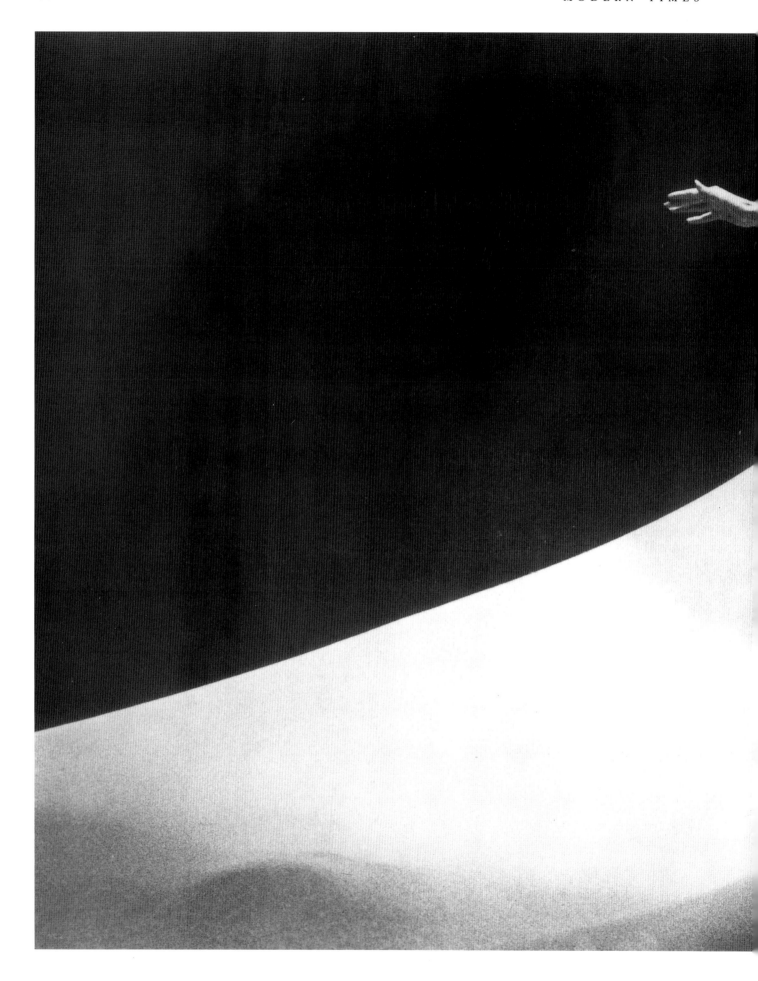

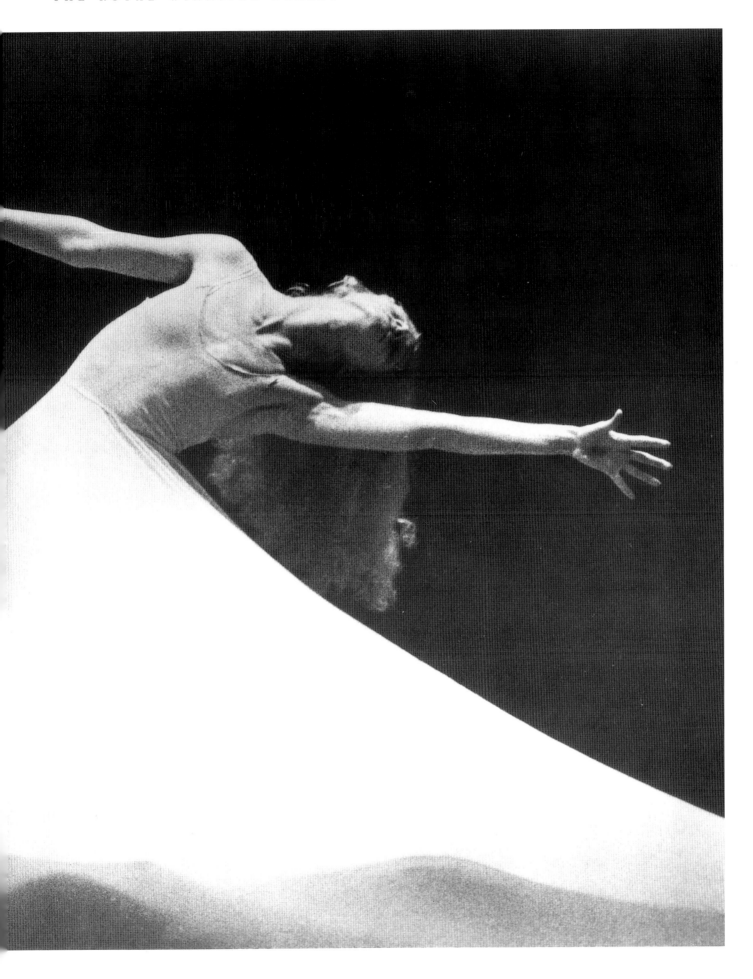

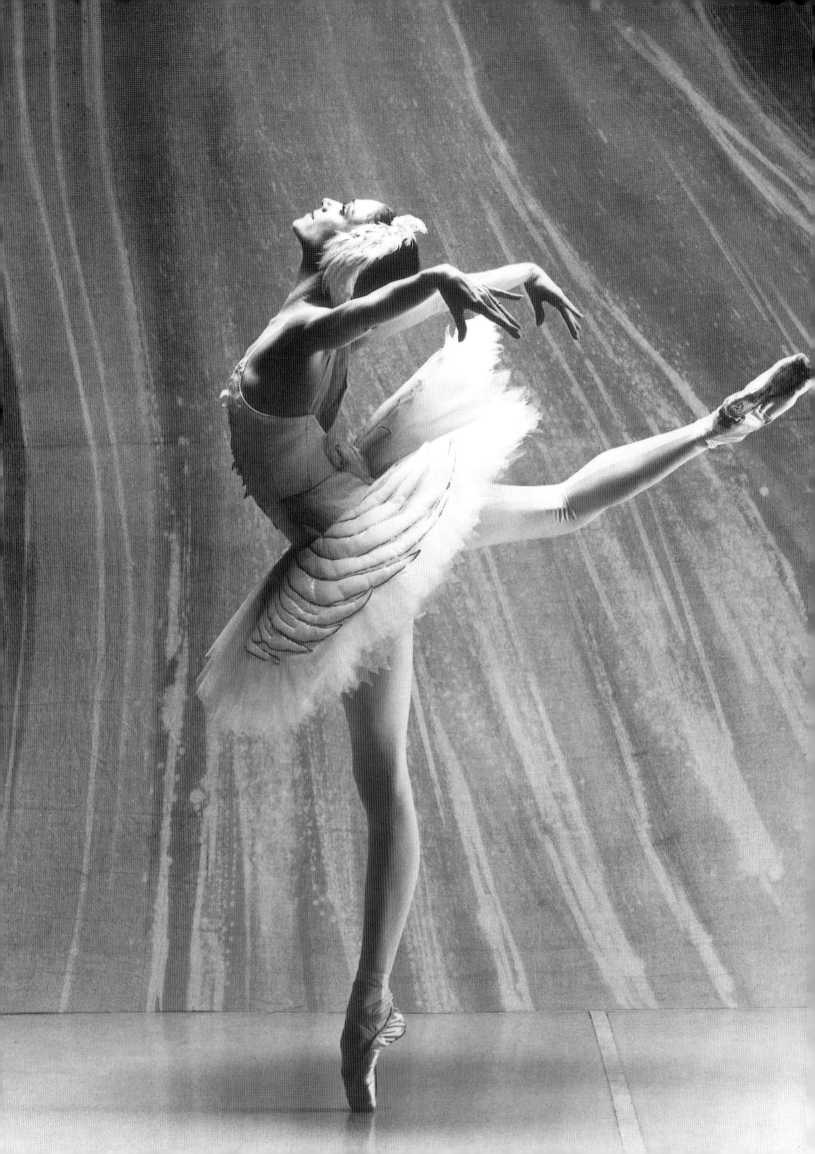

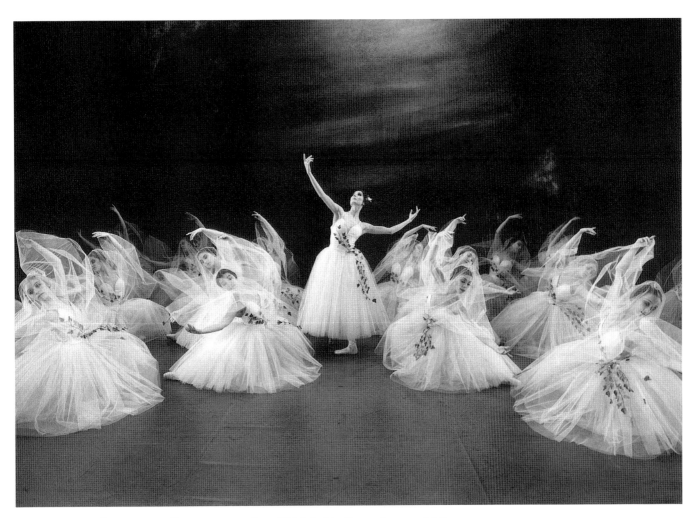

Facing page: Royal Winnipeg Ballet principal dancer Evelyn Hart, here as Odette in Galina Yordanova's 1987 production of *Swan Lake,* is regarded as one of the finest dancers ever produced in Canada. Trained in the professional division of the RWB school, she has won medals internationally and been acclaimed for her artistry throughout the world. (David Cooper photograph)

Peter Wright's *Giselle* was the second full-evening classic to enter the repertoire of the Royal Winnipeg Ballet, in 1984. Shown here: Patti Caplette as Myrthe, Queen of the Wilis, with the corps de ballet as the veiled spirits of jilted maidens. (David Cooper photograph)

Oscar Araiz's *Adagietto,* to a movement from Mahler's *Symphony No. 5,* entered the Royal Winnipeg Ballet repertoire in 1974. A popular pas de deux intended to depict "the changing of atmosphere from tenderness to ecstasy," it was danced in this 1978 casting by Bonnie Wyckoff and Joost Pelt. (Jack Mitchell photograph)

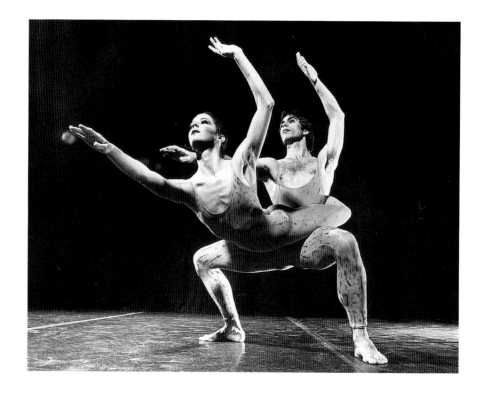

Norbert Vesak's *What to Do Till the Messiah Comes* was made for the Royal Winnipeg Ballet in 1973, to a collage of music by the rock groups Chilliwack and Syrinx and composer Phillip Werren. Shown is the 1978 cast (*left to right*): Bill Lark, Valerie Ford, Kathleen Duffy and Eric Horenstein. (Jack Mitchell photograph)

Facing page: Evelyn Hart and David Peregrine, two products of David Moroni's professional division of the Royal Winnipeg Ballet school, shot to international prominence after their successes at the Osaka and Varna festivals in 1980. Here they appear in the lead roles in the 1981 RWB production of Rudi van Dantzig's *Romeo and Juliet.* (David Cooper photograph)

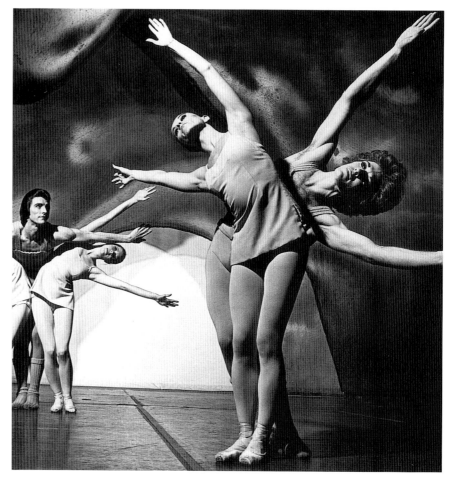

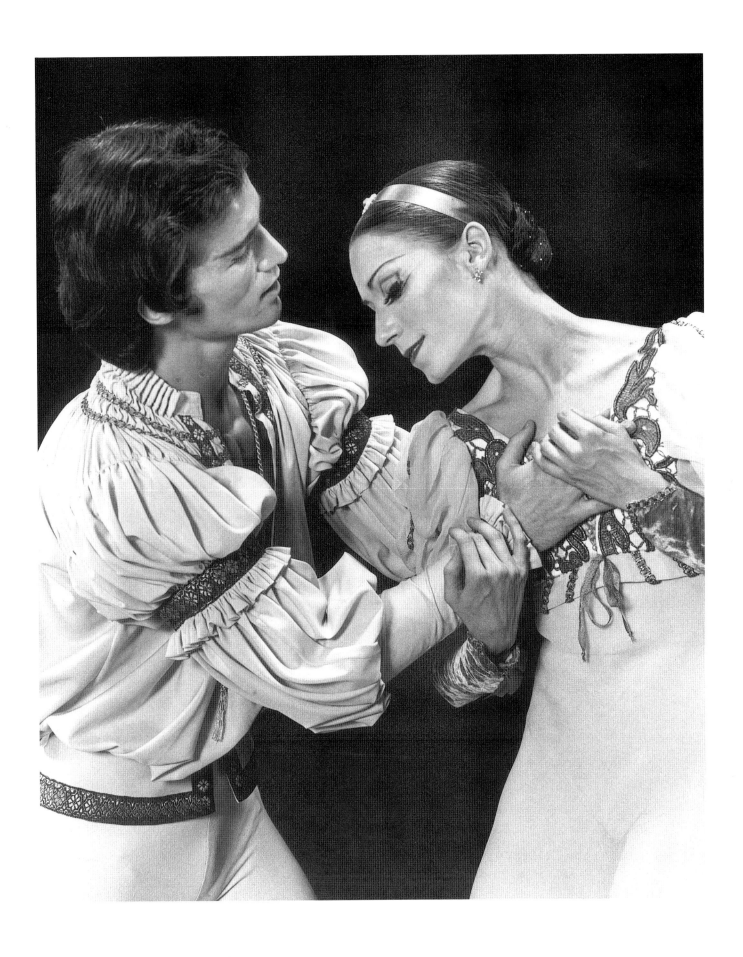

David Peregrine, shown here in Rudi van Dantzig's *Romeo and Juliet* with Royal Winnipeg Ballet partner Svea Eklof, died in 1989 when a light aircraft he was piloting crashed on a mountainside in Alaska. (David Cooper photograph)

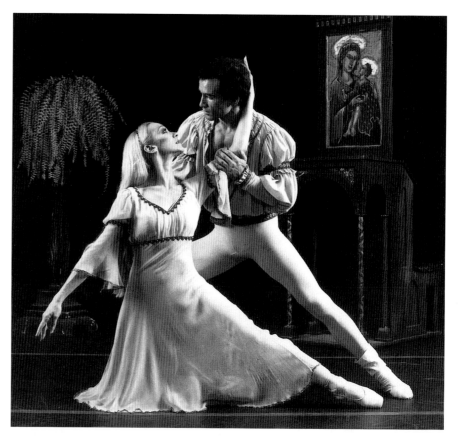

Theatre and dance designer Mary Kerr, composer Victor Davies and choreographer Jacques Lemay collaborated for the Royal Winnipeg Ballet's popular success, *The Big Top, a Circus Ballet,* in 1986. (David Cooper photograph)

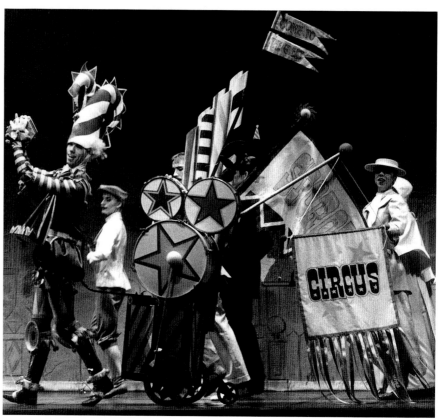

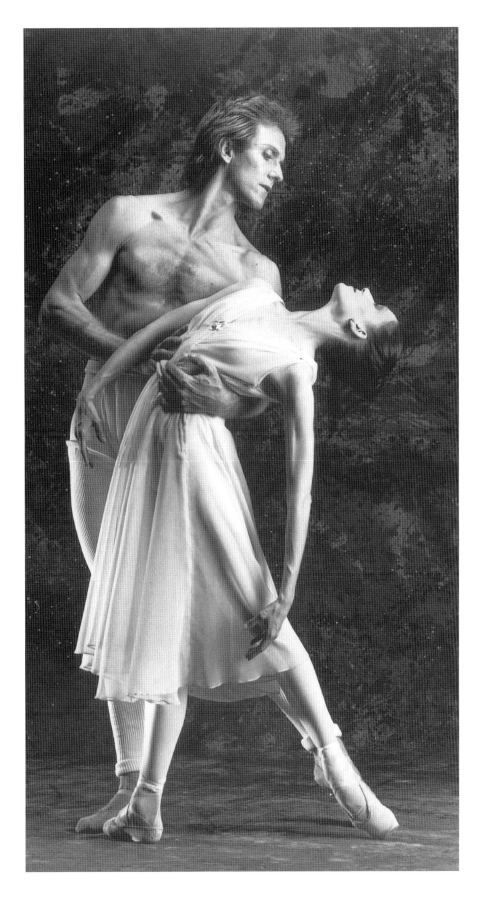

Hans van Manen's *Adagio Hammerklavier* was one of a number of works that displayed the partnership of the Royal Winnipeg Ballet's Evelyn Hart and Henny Jurriens during the late 1980s. Jurriens, a guest artist with the company from 1986, was artistic director for one season prior to his death in a road accident in April 1989. (David Cooper photograph)

Vincent Warren starred as Tommy, with
Hae Shik Kim as the Acid Queen, in
Fernand Nault's setting for Les Grands
Ballets Canadiens of the rock opera by
The Who. Repeatedly remounted, the
production was the economic salvation of
the company. (Courtesy Les Grands
Ballets Canadiens)

Facing page: Annette av Paul and
Alexandre Belin (also known as Sacha
Belinsky) in Brian Macdonald's *Au-delà
du temps* (*Time Out of Mind,*) a modern
fertility rite first made for New York's
Joffrey Ballet in 1963 and mounted on Les
Grands Ballets Canadiens a decade later.
(Courtesy Les Grands Ballets Canadiens)

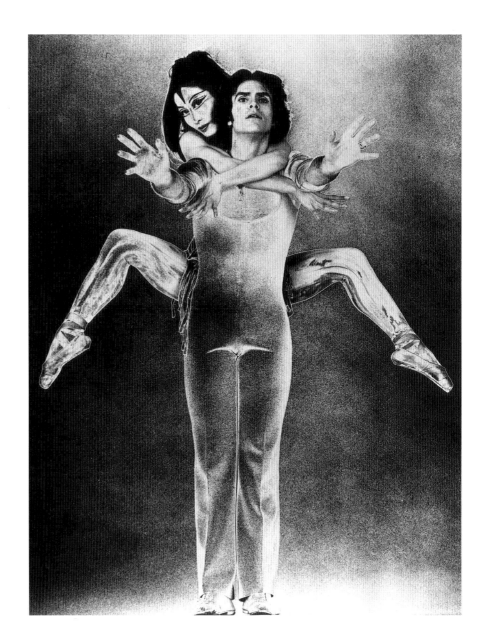

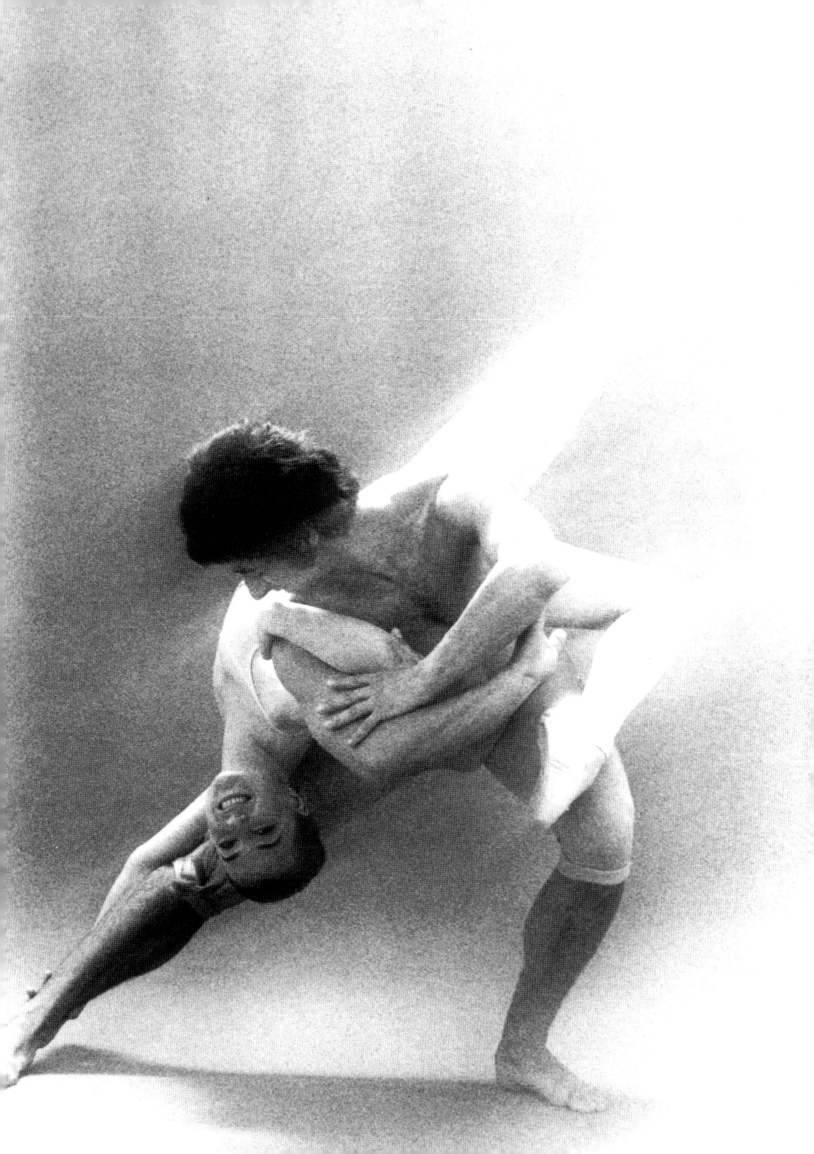

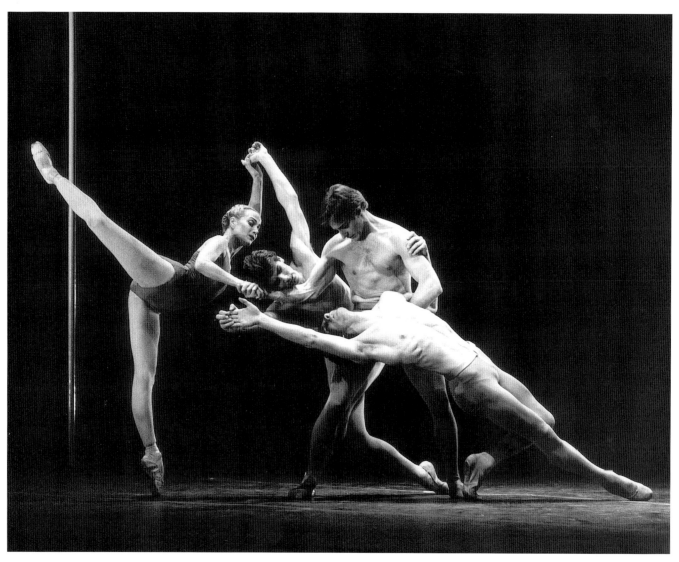

Brian Macdonald's *Double Quartet* was made for Les Grands Ballets Canadiens in 1978, and it is widely regarded as one of his most significant choreographic achievements. This photograph shows (*left to right*) Annette av Paul, Sylvain Senez, Jacques Drapeau and Sylvain Lafortune. (Melodie Garbish photograph)

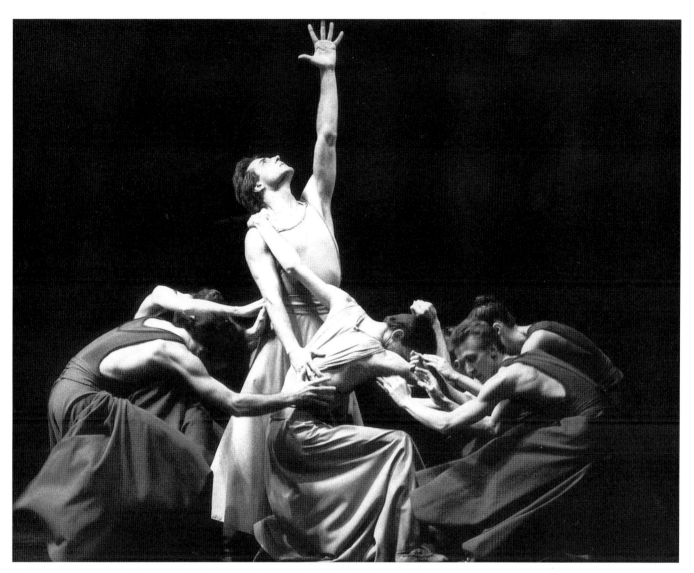

James Kudelka's *In Paradisum,* an elegiac, affecting discourse on loss and death, entered the repertoire of Les Grands Ballets Canadiens in 1983. It is regarded as one of Kudelka's most accomplished works. (Dominique Durocher photograph)

Overleaf: Serenade, a plotless, emotion-tinged ballet to music of Tchaikovsky, was the first work created by George Balanchine in North America, and remains one of his best loved and most widely performed. It entered the repertoire of Les Grands Ballets Canadiens in 1974. This shows a 1980 cast. (Andrew Oxenham photograph)

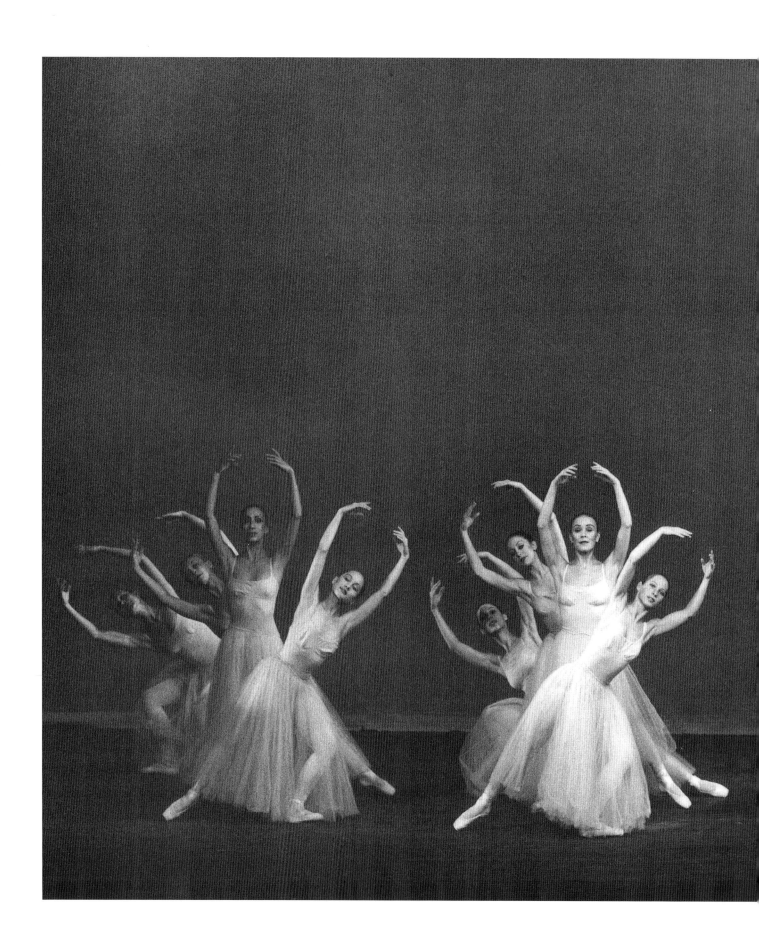

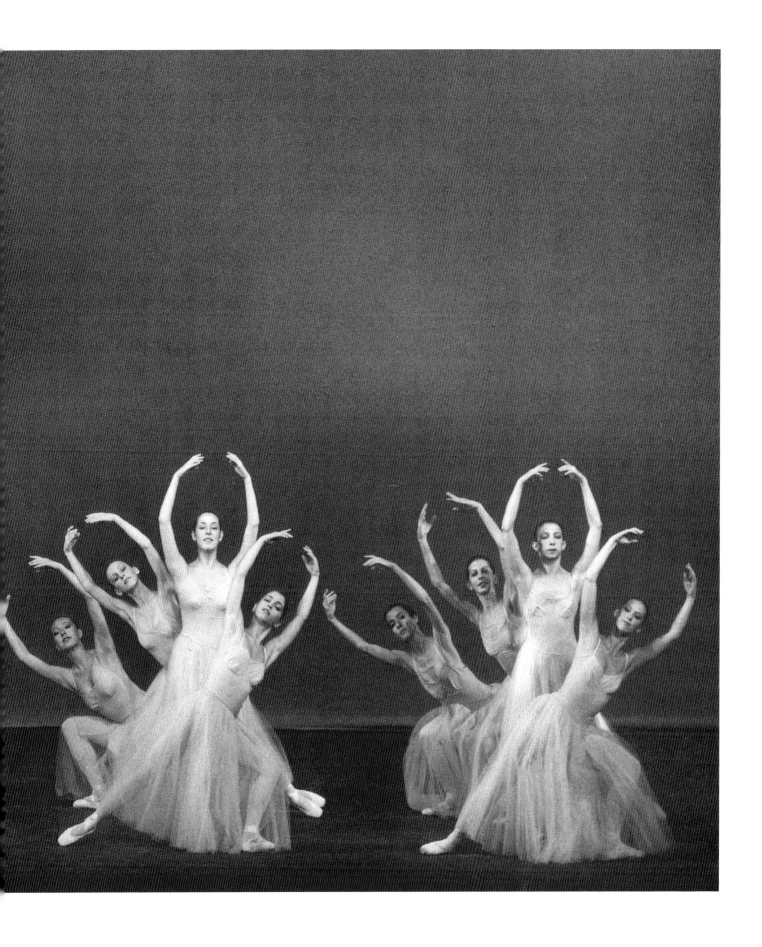

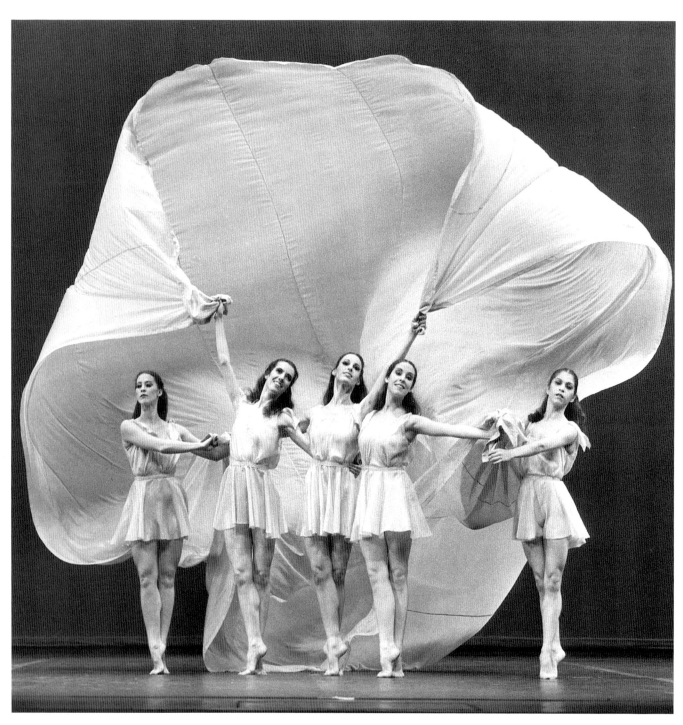

Soaring was one of the first works
choreographed by modern dance pioneer
Doris Humphrey, first performed in 1920
by the Ruth St. Denis Concert Dancers.
Recreated by Marion Rice, it entered the
repertoire of Les Grands Ballets
Canadiens in 1980. *Left to right:* Catherine
Lafortune, Josephine Baurac, Betsy
Baron, Hélène Grenier and Josée Ledoux.
(Andrew Oxenham photograph)

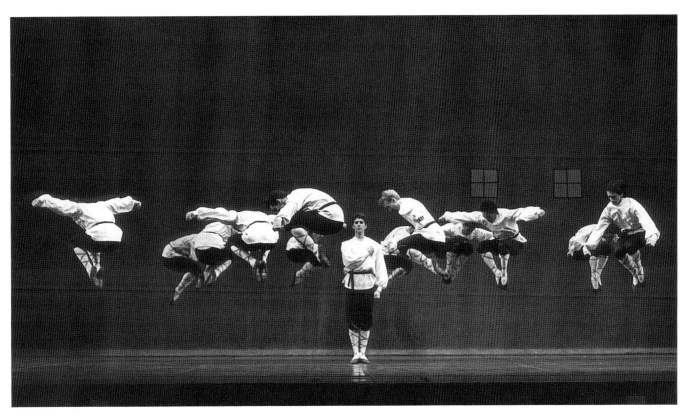

Bronislava Nijinska's *Les Noces,* an evocation of peasant wedding rites in Russia, was first performed by the Diaghilev Ballets Russes in Paris in 1923. It was staged for Les Grands Ballets Canadiens in the 1986–87 season. Shown here are Sylvain Senez and male company members. (Andrew Oxenham photograph)

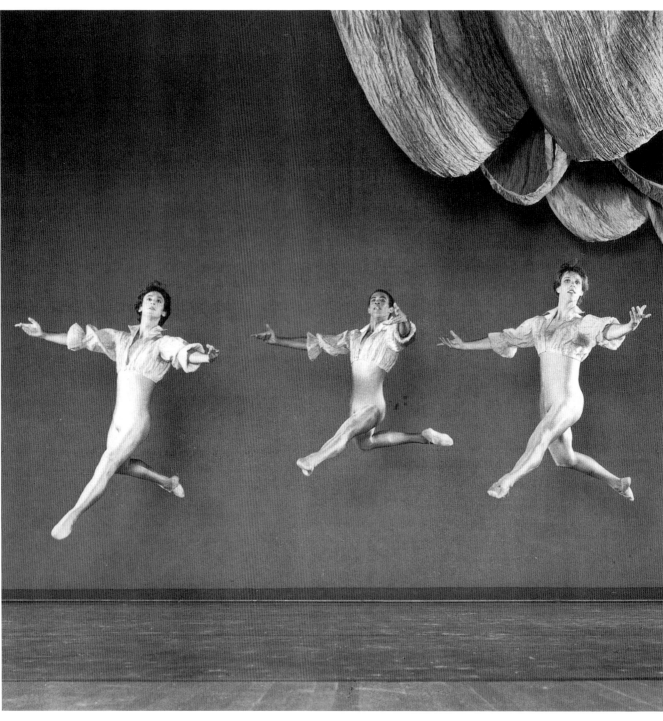

Lawrence Gradus made *Tribute* for Theatre Ballet of Canada in 1981 in memory of Jacqueline Lemieux, his wife and his collaborator in the creation of Entre-Six. The work became a Theatre Ballet signature-piece. (Ken Bell photograph)

Facing page: The Creation of Eve, made by Renald Rabu for Pacific Ballet Theatre in 1981, was inspired by a print by B.C. artist Roy Vickers, telling the Eden story in the style of Pacific Northwest Coast Indian art. Vickers also designed and painted the costumes, worn here by Charie Evans and

Gaetan Masse. (Rodney Polden Photographics)

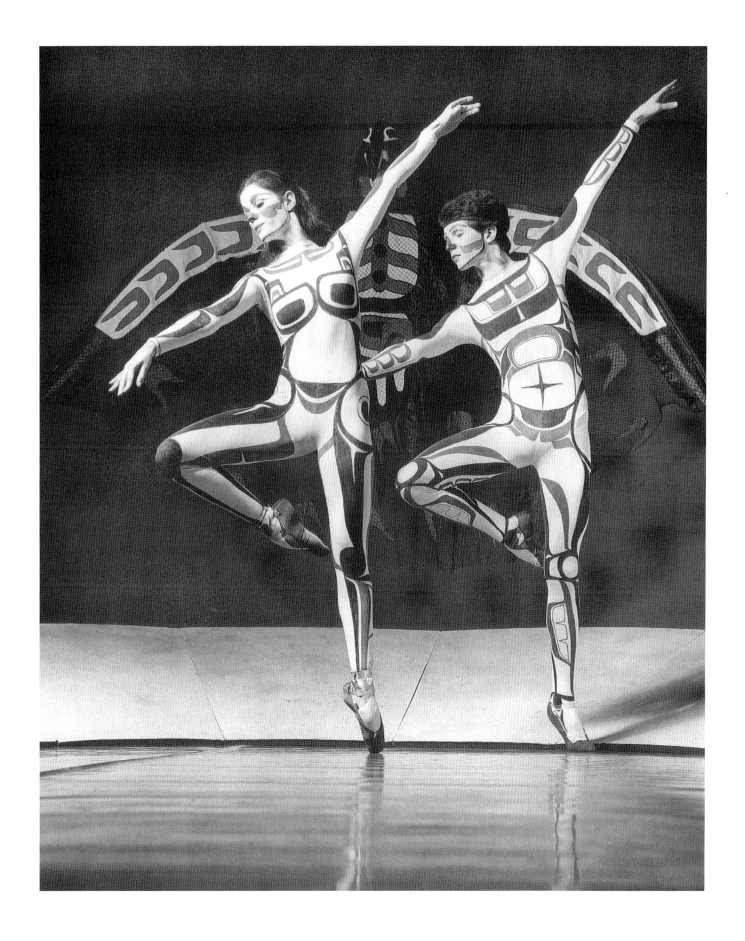

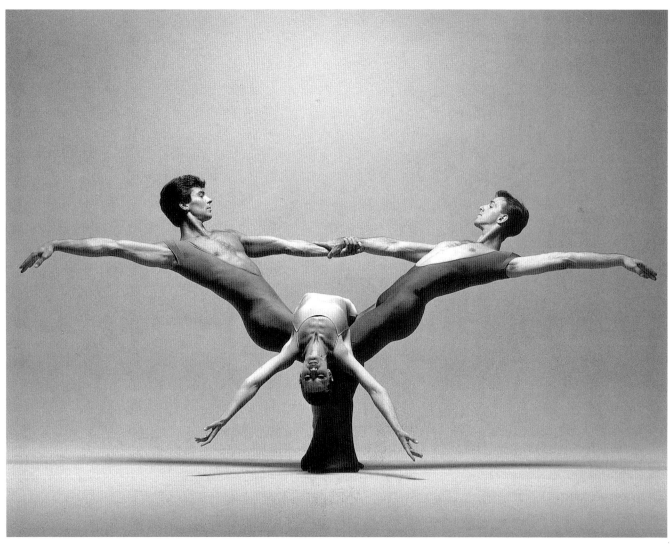

Czech-born, Holland-based choreographer Jiri Kylian's *Return to the Strange Land* was one of a group of works chosen by Ballet British Columbia's Reid Anderson to help define the lean, European style he began to forge for the company during his period as artistic director from 1987 to 1989. *Left to right:* David MacGillivray, Charie Evans and Bernard Sauvé. (David Cooper photograph)

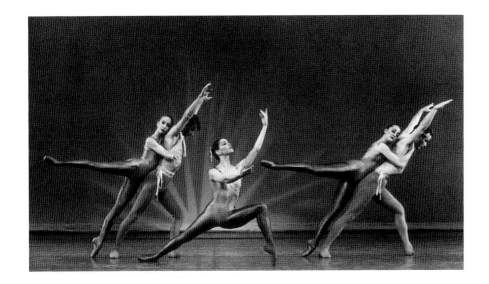

Lambros Lambrou made *Sundances* in 1979 for the Alberta Ballet, where he was resident choreographer. The light, popular work, which uses the classical language with an accent reflecting Lambrou's Greek heritage, subsequently entered the repertoire of many companies, among them the Royal Winnipeg Ballet. (Ed Ellis photograph)

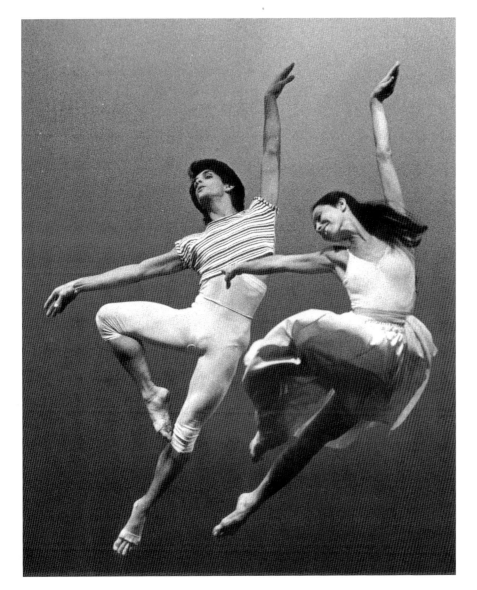

Five New Waves, by U.S. choreographer Rael Lamb, entered the repertoire of Montreal's Les Ballets Jazz in the late 1970s, along with a range of specifically created jazz-dance works by other U.S. and Canadian choreographers. Pictured are Jacques Marcil and Anne Barlett. (Andrew Oxenham photograph)

Modern Dance

TORONTO: *The Hothouse*

The upheavals that shook the National Ballet of Canada in the early 1970s materially influenced the development of Canadian modern dance. Out of the protected conservatory of professional ballet and into the wide-open field of modern dance popped three individuals who, in very different ways, were to help shape the future of choreographic creativity in the country—Grant Strate and Lawrence and Miriam Adams.

Strate had spent 20 often difficult years with the National. What was needed, he believed, was a climate in which individual creativity could grow, free of the immediate need to satisfy an audience. So in 1971 he quit the company and took a post that would allow him to create that climate—founding chairman of the dance department at York University. The programme he evolved provided the kind of training that individuals previously had to travel to New York to find. It was the country's first centralized base for a full range of modern techniques, and while it included options in areas like notation, dance therapy, history and criticism, its focus was on equipping individuals for survival as professional dancers. Its graduates were to find work in virtually every modernist company in the country; some launched successful companies of their own.

But Strate's influence on dance creativity in Canada did not stop at York. In 1978 and again in 1980 he organized national choreographic seminars in which young choreographers spent a month teamed with composers in a programme constructed to force creative risk. The experience "opened up avenues I scarcely dreamed were at my disposal," said James Kudelka, reminiscing about the 1980 seminar for *Dance in Canada* magazine.

In 1980 Strate moved to Simon Fraser University in British Columbia, where, as director of the Centre for the Arts, he continued to release onto the national dance scene a steady stream of innovative creators.

———

Lawrence Adams and his wife Miriam Weinstein, a member of the corps, left the National Ballet in 1970, tired of what they felt was a stifled and stifling routine. The following year they and some friends launched a company called 15 Dancers (because that's how many they were) and toured an eclectic experimental repertoire. A typical evening might include a jazz solo, a pessimistic statement about alienation, a video experiment and a duet by Miriam on the theme of yoghurt.

In early 1973 the company, now down to five, turned a former enamel-baking shop in downtown Toronto into a 52-seat theatre and presented a new show every weekend. Once, the show consisted of Lawrence building a brick wall. Another time it was the 15 Dancers' *Nutcracker*, a full-length spoof by a cast of four; they asked the Canada Council for a $300 grant to finance the production, and got it.

In the fall of 1974 the Adamses gave up performing, named the space 15 Dance Laboratorium, and threw open its doors. They called it their *atelier*; they called themselves the janitors. The young experimenters flocked. By this time, the New York experimentalist movement was well established. Post-modernism in dance had begun with an informal group of choreographers who gathered at the Judson Church in 1962. They pushed Merce Cunningham's assertion that movement could exist of itself to new extremes. Spontaneous activity won new significance; so did contact improvisation, an improvised interaction for two or more.

Lawrence and Miriam Adams subsequently claimed they had little knowledge of the New York experimentalist movement when they set up 15 Dance Laboratorium. "We were hothousing," said Lawrence, "force-growing some kind of rapid escalation in dance activity in the city."

A $5,000 Ontario Arts Council grant underwrote the first season. Dancers who took part (many of them graduates from Strate's programme at York) included three of the trailblazers of the Canadian independent-choreographer movement: Anna Blewchamp, Judy Jarvis and Jennifer Mascall, all of whom subsequently won national choreographic awards. In all, 135 choreographers played the Lab in the six years it was open, drawing audiences that ranged in number from 3 to 90.

In the mid-1970s, people used to joke that every time a York University dance department class graduated, five new dance companies were formed. One of the most enduring was Dancemakers, founded by a pair of York graduates, Andrea Ciel Smith and Marcy Radler, in 1974. At the time of its launching, it was the only modern dance company in Toronto apart from Toronto Dance Theatre, and established itself as a company of unpretentious seriousness and cool wit, with an international and eclectic repertoire emphasizing technique, form and accessibility rather than outrageous experiment.

It subsequently went through regular changes of leading personnel. Peggy Smith Baker and Patricia Miner became co-directors for the 1977–78 season, were succeeded by Anna Blewchamp, then Baker took over for a further year. In 1980 Carol Anderson, one of the company's founding members, and Patricia Fraser became co-artistic directors, with Anderson assuming sole charge in 1985 and remaining as resident choreographer when Bill James took control in 1988.

Toronto Independent Dance Enterprise (TIDE) was founded in 1978 by a group of York graduates as a collective co-operative for dancers, choreographers and composers. For some years it operated around a nucleus of four dancer-choreographers—Paula Ravitz, Allan Risdill, Sallie Lyons and Denise Fujiwara—creating from a mixture of traditional technique, gesture and contact improvisation a body of work that, in its gritty unsentimentality, its of-the-moment spontaneity and its consistent imaginative daring, stood at the forefront of experimentalism in Canada. Eventually, sole control of the company passed to Fujiwara.

It was a single work, made at York University in 1975, that led to the creation of the Danny Grossman Dance Company. Grossman grew up in a strongly politicized household in San Francisco and danced as a principal for more than a decade with Paul Taylor's company in New York. His connections with Toronto

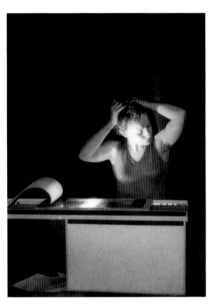

Elizabeth Chitty was one of many performance experimenters who honed their art at Toronto's 15 Dance Laboratorium in the 1970s. In this 1978 photograph, she performs her work Demo Model. *(Zontal photograph)*

dated back to 1962, when he met Toronto Dance Theatre's David Earle at the American Dance Festival at Connecticut College. In 1973 Earle invited Grossman to guest with the company for three weeks; the three weeks became a season, and eventually Grossman settled permanently in the city.

His first venture into choreography, the graceful and athletic balancing act *Higher*, made at York in 1975, was taken into the TDT repertoire and became his signature piece. In 1978 he founded his own professional company. Its repertoire is built on extended explorations of his personal style—staccato, witty, athletic, exuberant. The social concerns are never far away—the spoofing of empty patriot gesture in *National Spirit*, the threat to humanity posed by war in *Endangered Species*, the sombre religious penitents of *Ecce Homo*—but his choreography also displays (echoes of Taylor) a concern with pure energy, a sense of wry fun and witty frolic, an angular disjointedness, an arresting physicality and sense of danger.

Grossman was one of two Toronto modernists invited by Erik Bruhn to work with the National Ballet of Canada in the mid-1980s. The other was Robert Desrosiers, a former National Ballet dancer who had performed in France, England (with the Lindsay Kemp experimental mime-dance-theatre company) and in Canada before establishing his own troupe in 1980. He has been acclaimed internationally for the extravagance, audacity and brilliance of his theatrical imagination, less so for his choreography. Although the movement content itself was often thin and limited, he created (in works like the National Ballet commission, *Blue Snake*, with its monster-head that gobbled up dancers, or in rich imaginative explosions like *L'Hôtel perdu*, in which a pianist in full formal dress carried a grand piano on his back) physical theatre of a romantic neosurrealism that, in its extravagance and flamboyant colorations, was utterly of its time.

Lawrence and Miriam Adams, meanwhile, launched a brief-lived national monthly, *Canadian Dance News*, after the closure of 15 Dance Lab in 1980, and in 1982 initiated Encore! Encore!, a research organization devoted to the preservation of Canadian dance history. It established a Dance Hall of Fame and in 1986 brought together a group of dance pioneers to reconstruct and tape six "lost" Canadian ballets from the 1930s and 1940s.

An interesting historical throwback in Toronto modern dance at this time was the work of Judy Jarvis, a choreographer active from about 1970. She had spent three years in Germany studying with Mary Wigman, and was Canada's most direct link with German expressionism, working in a simple and direct choreographic style.

———

Establishment modern dance in Toronto fared less well than the experimenters. Toronto Dance Theatre suffered setback after setback in the 1970s, culminating in a mass resignation in 1980 (four dancers and most of the administrative staff) and, in 1981, removal of its operating-grant status with the Canada Council.

The company was in crisis. It was hard to define—creative crucible, international touring company, theatre collaborative, what? And it had come to be regarded as a haven of dance conservatism. The three directors were the rocks on which the company had been built; they were the rocks on which it now came close to foundering.

It took two outsiders to sort the situation out. Ed Oscapella, a concert agent, became company administrator late in 1981, and turned around the financing. And in 1983 Kenny Pearl, a Canadian who had spent a decade in New York dancing with the Martha Graham and Alvin Ailey companies, was appointed artistic director, removing the pressure from the three founders, who became (along with brilliant company alumnus Christopher House) resident choreographers.

Within a year, what David Earle had termed a nightmare became a reawakening and revitalization of the company. By 1985, *New York Times* critic Anna Kisselgoff (reserving special praise for the "kinetic brilliance" of the "downright startling" choreography of Christopher House) was writing: "The company is good, disciplined, and one to watch in the future."

Pearl left the company in the fall of 1987, and David Earle, refreshed and ready to reassume responsibility, became sole artistic director, with Beatty, Randazzo and House alongside him as resident choreographers and Ken Peirson as administrative director. In its twentieth anniversary season, 1988–89, the company was as active, in terms of numbers of performances across the country, as the National Ballet of Canada.

SMALLER HOTBEDS EVERYWHERE

The dance explosion of the late 1960s and early 1970s forced a host of small modern-dance companies of mixed technical persuasions and varying durability through the Canadian permafrost.

Principal among the new modernist growth in Vancouver was the Anna Wyman Dance Theatre, founded in 1971. Born in Graz, Austria, Anna Wyman began her dancing career in ballet but later, under the influence of the movement theories of Rudolf von Laban, turned to modern dance. She studied, taught and choreographed in London before moving to Vancouver in 1967, and launched her company, initially a performing ensemble of advanced students, in 1971. It turned professional in 1973, and that year travelled to the International Young Choreographers' Competition in Cologne, Germany, where her work *Here at the Eye of the Hurricane* was chosen as one of the three best works on display. In 1975 the company undertook the first national tour by a modern-dance troupe and has since toured extensively around the world. In 1980 it was the first modern dance company from the West to tour China. The performance style was initially based on spontaneous creativity; it evolved into an extended exploration of linearity and geometrics, and later relaxed into a warmer, more romantic feel. Anna Wyman's intense theatricality, and her use of props and technological aids like film and lasers, earned comparisons with New York's Alwin Nikolais.

The federal government's make-work programmes of the early 1970s, the Local Initiatives Programme and Opportunities for Youth, encouraged the emergence of new groups in all the performing arts.

In Vancouver, two of the more durable dance products of these programmes were Prism Dance Theatre (launched as Contemporary-Jazz Dance Theatre in

1973 by Jamie Zagoudakis, and directed by Zagoudakis and Gisa Cole until it closed in the mid-1980s) and Mountain Dance Theatre (a 1973 spin-off from a summer course at Simon Fraser University, initially directed by Mauryne Allan and Freddie Long, run by Allan alone from 1979 to its disappearance in 1987 and reincarnated as Dancecorps in 1988 with Cornelius Fischer-Credo as artistic director).

Also active in Vancouver from 1973 to 1976 was Tournesol, which claimed to be Canada's smallest dance company (two, Ernst Eder and his wife Carole) and set out to "reflect the state of being of the dance couple living, teaching, performing and choreographing as a unit."

But the Vancouver company with the most far-reaching effect on the development of new dance thinking in the city was Terminal City Dance, another enterprise that had its roots in Iris Garland's dance programme at Simon Fraser University. It began in 1974 as a collaboration between teacher Karen Rimmer (a former SFU student who had been a member of the Alwin Nikolais company in New York) and student Savannah Walling, who had also studied at the Nikolais studio and had become interested in mime. They did a joint concert of choreography that fall, were joined by three other dancers for a nine-month experimental dance workshop in 1975, and gave their first performance under the name of Terminal City Dance in 1976.

The company reconstituted itself from year to year, always around a basic core of three (Rimmer, Walling and Terry Hunter, another former mime), and by the early 1980s was presenting works which displayed an evolving movement language that integrated dance, music and theatre in startling ways. In 1982, the partnership broke up. The following year, Walling and Hunter adopted the name Special Delivery Dance/Music/Theatre, to indicate the directions in which they planned to move their work, and Rimmer, reverting to her maiden name, formed her own troupe, the Karen Jamieson Dance Company.

Walling and Hunter embarked on a search for a theatricality of movement that went beyond the boundaries of Western dance, using mime, mask, percussion, voice, clowning and fantastical myth-characters in an effort to discover and express what Hunter called "an energy, a spirit, a consciousness which is common to all human heritage."

Jamieson, meanwhile, set out on a search for the same universality of emotional and intellectual metaphor, but within the broad Western dance-theatre tradition. Works like *Coming Out of Chaos* (about the challenges faced by man, a small scrap at the mercy of large forces, in his attempts to realize his potential), *Sisyphus* (to do with human indomitability in the face of impossible odds) and *Rainforest* (a fusion of post-modern dance techniques with traditional West Coast Indian myth and image-making) tried to extend the communicative possibilities of human movement by the creation of an uncluttered manner of expression that strikes direct to the emotions or the viscera. It was a direct connection back to the animating principles of the early modern dancers of the U.S. and their attempts to project dramatic content in an abstract way through a controlled choreographic language.

Deliberately distancing herself from modernism's cutting edge is another Vancouver-based choreographer, Judith Marcuse. Born in Montreal, she trained

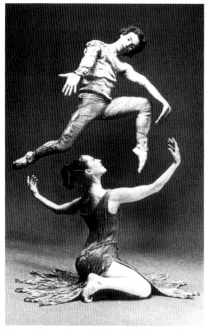

Maria Formolo and Keith Urban perform Renaissance, *a suite of six lively dances for two, to music of Toronto composer Srul Irving Glick, created by Urban in 1980 for Regina Modern Dance Works. (Frank Richards photograph)*

initially with her aunt, Elsie Salomons, and with the early European modernist Seda Zaré, before moving to London's Royal Ballet School and embarking on a career as a professional dancer with companies in Switzerland, Israel, the U.S. and London. She began to choreograph while working with the Ballet Rambert in London, but was not known as a choreographer in Canada until Brian Macdonald invited her to make a work for Les Grands Ballets. She settled in Vancouver in 1976 and established a company four years later. Her personal performance style—a kind of fluid anger, a compacted aggression, emotionally loaded—won her wide acclaim; she was the first artist to win Canada's two principal choreographic prizes. Her choreography, a securely structured language of ballet-tinged modern movement, displays a similar commitment—a devotion to dancing that is done full-out, with a flung and sometimes angry passion; a determination never merely to doodle in space; a celebration of the sexuality of movement. Although her company's repertoire emphasizes the work of Marcuse, it also features a broad spectrum of dance by Canadian and international choreographers.

There have been several attempts to establish professional modern dance on the prairies.

In Edmonton, where modern dance activity dates back to Dorothy Harris's first course in creative dance at the University of Alberta in 1952, the Alberta Contemporary Dancers was launched in 1971 by Jacqueline Ogg and Charlene Tarver, but collapsed in financial disarray in 1978. It was succeeded in 1979 by the Brian Webb Dance Company, based at Grant MacEwan College.

In Calgary, the two-man theatre-dance troupe Sun*Ergos has been operated by Dana Luebke and Robert Greenwood since 1977. Two years later, Elaine Bowman, a modern dance instructor at the University of Calgary, and Peter Hoff launched Dancers' Studio West, the chief champion of professional modern dance in the city.

Regina Modern Dance Works evolved from a workshop created by Marianne Livant, a former member of the Ann Arbor Dance Theatre, who arrived in Canada in 1967. In 1974 she teamed up with another American, Maria Formolo, and Susan Jane Arnold, both formerly with Le Groupe de la Place Royale, to launch a professional company. Philosophical differences soon split the group, and Formolo ran the company alone for several years before joining up with former Toronto Dance Theatre dancer Keith Urban in 1979. In 1982 they moved moved to Edmonton as Urban and Formolo Dance, and in 1985 Formolo established herself as a solo artist.

In the eastern and western extremes of Canada, modern dance has been sparsely represented. In Victoria, B.C., David Dressler was teaching experimental movement and body therapy from 1973, but the city's only successful professional company was Spectrum Dance Circus, founded in 1978 by a former New Yorker, Constantine Darling (also director of a Montreal jazz-dance company, Shango Dance Theatre, from 1972 to 1975). It closed in 1986. Active in Victoria since that time as a solo artist is former Paula Ross and Spectrum dancer Lynda Raino.

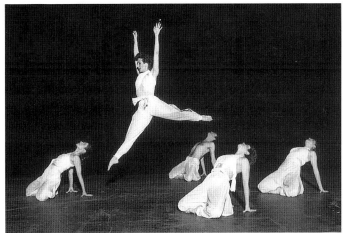

Grecia was created for Nova Dance Theatre in Halifax by Jeanne Robinson in 1985. Left to right: *Pat Cloutis, Leica Hardy, Cliff LeJeune, Christiane Miron and Suzanne Miller. (Greg McKinnon photograph)*

The first modern dance company in Prince Edward Island was the Island Dance Ensemble, formed in 1975 by Sekai (formerly Blaine Vany) and Joy Jackson. Sekai moved to Halifax in 1977 to work with the Halifax Dance Co-op, which had been set up as an umbrella organization and informal company in 1973, and that fall created Sekai and Company. He moved to Montreal in 1979, and in 1981 a former member of his Halifax company, Jeanne Robinson, established Nova Dance Theatre, a professional company based in Halifax. Nova survived until 1987.

Other amateur and semiprofessional modernist troupes that have had varying success in the Maritime provinces include Montage Dance Theatre in Charlottetown, P.E.I., the Newfoundland Dance Theatre in St. John's, and DansEncorps and DancEast in Moncton, New Brunswick.

QUEBEC: Overleaping the Bounds

The new courage and sense of cultural pride felt by the Québécois after the "quiet revolution" of 1960 permeated every level of Quebec society. Film-makers began to find lasting significance in Quebec subjects and themes. Michel Tremblay's 1968 play, Les Belles-Soeurs, brought joual, the dialect of the common people, to the stage for the first time. Through television, singers like Robert Charlebois and Pauline Julien spread the message of Québécois dignity and identity; the very act of creating became a political gesture. In dance, the change could be seen in the new freedom that was abroad—a freedom that Quebec, with all its historical baggage, perhaps felt even more acutely than the rest of Canada. In the late 1970s and early 1980s there was extended exploration in the Montreal choreographic community of three topics that had been off-limits—sex, politics and the church.

One of the most significant influences on the emerging Montreal dance scene in terms of inspiration to experiment was Le Groupe de la Place Royale, founded in 1966. In 1969 Canada Council support was withdrawn abruptly after an unfortunate outburst in print by Peter Boneham (he accused the council of trying to kill modern dance), and in 1971, Jeanne Renaud—who had initially provided most of the choreography, a kind of kinetic intellectualizing, disciplined, clear, austere, with a strong sense of line and design—decided she had had enough. She was exhausted by the constant battles over money, and she and Boneham had reached a philosophic parting of the ways.

Boneham assumed control of the company, with Jean-Pierre Perreault, then one of the company's leading dancers, as his artistic assistant, and in 1977 they moved to Ottawa, complaining volubly about Quebec's lack of policy, criteria or priorities for dance support. Grants, said Perreault, were simply being marketed to suit public taste. Two years later, the Quebec ministry of culture established a bureau to deal specifically with dance. At its head was Jeanne Renaud.

Martine Epoque's Groupe Nouvelle Aire, which offered its first public performances in the spring of 1971, became a forcing-house for a generation of choreographers that changed the face of dance in Canada.

The group had its origins as a research unit in Epoque's dance programme at the University of Montreal's physical education department. To make dancers out of gymnasts who had no previous dance technique, Epoque invented a style of her own based on principles of anatomy and eurhythmics. The group's earliest choreographic imprint was a rhythmic, sharp-edged linearity, though this was gradually to change, like that of Le Groupe de la Place Royale, to a fluid expressiveness more in tune with the neoromantic times.

The company never achieved the prominence enjoyed by Le Groupe de la Place Royale, but it was Nouvelle Aire that was responsible for the return to choreography of Françoise Sullivan, and it was at Nouvelle Aire's studios that a core of dancers who contributed to the explosion of independent choreographic activity in Montreal in the late 1970s and 1980s cut their first choreographic teeth.

One of the first was Paul-André Fortier, who set up as an independent in 1979 and established a formal company under his own name in 1981. His early work was characteristic of the Québécois artist's deep, questioning involvement with the newly emerging Quebec society—forceful, even violent in its imagery, infused with an intense sexuality and a theatricality that was at times as simplistic and direct as a political broadside. In *Violence* a red garden hose became a monstrous phallus and chief weapon in a male-female struggle for domination. *Fin* was one of a number of works in which he used rocks as symbols of life's responsibilities and the need for the individual to conform.

Later works were more subtle and more complex, though their attack on the social jugular remained as violent. At the same time, there was always an undertow of humanity, a wry hope; his work was an early precursor of the neoromantic, neo-expressionist dance theatricality that typified new dance in Montreal in the 1980s.

The movement he used had none of the expected gestural qualities of established modern dance. Raw and primal, it was often a matter of pushed-forward pelvises and draped-back shoulders, of angular, roosterlike elbows and knees. His dancers strutted and staggered, writhed and hobbled, shuffled and skipped.

There were reasons for this technical primitivism. The seminal modern-dance movement of America had left no mark on the new generation of Montreal makers of new dance. The city had never been able to support sustained teaching in formal modern styles. Instead, what Montreal developed, uniquely in Canada, was a generation of choreographers with no foundations in the modernist traditions—but with saturation exposure to the generation of New York *post*-modernists, in particular, the Judson Church experimenters who had moved on from Cunningham to strip away the trappings conventionally associated with theatre-dance: beauty, technique, structure, meaning, even theatrical space itself.

This exposure was provided principally through the activities of choreographer Dena Davida and an artist-run space called Tangente: danse actuelle that Davida established in 1979 as a showcase for both U.S. and Canadian independents. In the late 1970s and early 1980s she introduced Montreal audiences to virtually all the post-modernist ground-breakers; in 1983 she organized a New York–Montreal "dance exchange," with seven Canadians sharing four weekends of programmes with eight New Yorkers.

Fortier won the Chalmers award in 1981. The following year it went to Edouard

Lock, another Nouvelle Aire alumnus but, in terms of style and effect, a descendant both of post-modernist New York and of the new theatricalized expressionism that was emerging in German modern dance.

And it was now that Canadian modernism began to pick up the threads of the European influence again. The tradition of psychological expressiveness that had made European dance so unfashionable when the modernists and post-modernists were beginning to dominate dance in America now reasserted itself. This time, however, it was no longer a matter of the wholesale importation of style, but a healthier selectiveness of influence. Some of the most interesting developments in experimentalist choreography in Canada had to do with the attempted integration of the various innovations of New York with the advances made by Europe's neo-expressionists in the areas of narrative, emotion and psychological insight.

In Lock's theatre-pieces the sexual interplay of power was examined in close-up, at its most physical. His choreography, dense, spasmic and obsessively frenzied, was deeply rooted in risk. Sometimes his dancers threw themselves in splayed, backward leaps through the air, or flew sideways as if some unseen hand had yanked them by the shoulder. Sometimes other dancers threw them; sometimes they seemed to explode from repose into airborne starbursts. Lead dancer Louise Lecavalier often appeared wearing a small, blonde moustache, and the dancers regularly took equal shares of the physical burdens and risks. Their mid-flight intertwining and thumping crashes declared not just a joyous independence but a tough love. It was also an exercise in the manipulation of style and art, blending the fashionable physical theatrics of the day with an attenuated post-punk sensibility. With their fast-cut, meticulously orchestrated visual attack, their live, loud, ingratiating techno-pop music, Lock's dances were like elongated rock videos, and their punk appeal embraced both the rock audience and the alternative-gallery crowd. In 1988 he collaborated with rock singer David Bowie on a London stage presentation that one British journalist called "the best seven minutes I've ever seen."

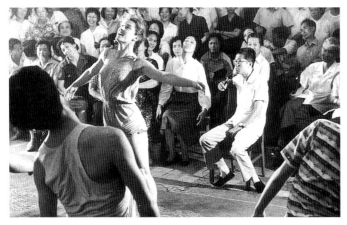

The individual's response to social pressure remained a recurrent theme in Québécois new dance throughout the 1980s. "All our dances are political," said Daniel Léveillé, another Nouvelle Aire alumnus who was active as an independent in the early 1980s. "We are the voice of Quebec, and we hope others will follow. But dance is universal, and we can see the problems of the world."

As the social outfall of Quebec's cultural revolution began to settle and the political involvement of the artistic community began to lessen, the outlines of other schools began to emerge—choreographers more interested in form than content, choreographers more interested in ritual than message.

Montreal modernist Margie Gillis gives a class for the Beijing Ballet during her visit to China in 1979. Gillis, who says she regards dancing as "a possibility for requited love," captivated the Chinese with her freestyle emotional outpourings on the stage. (Jack Udashkin photograph)

Linda Rabin, a Montreal-born choreographer who danced in Israel and Britain before settling in Montreal in 1975, was one who emphasized form. Trained in the José Limón technique, she created works for Les Grands Ballets and a number of modernist groups as well as for her own Triskelian Dance Foundation. In dance that celebrated the craft of movement, the structures of music and the uncomplicated pleasures of dancing, she established herself as an exponent of dynamic modern classicism, offering unsentimental, uncosmeticized dance-making that hinted, in its severe, nonliteral manner, at the austere, abstract beauties of the great neoclassicist of the ballet, George Balanchine.

One of the chief ritualists was Françoise Sullivan, who returned to choreography in 1977 as part of a Nouvelle Aire workshop that featured contributions from the "older generation" of Montreal choreographers: Sullivan, Renaud, Riopelle, Chiriaeff, Salomons and Nault. Sullivan's seven-hour session included a revival of *Dédale*, an arm-swinging solo from 1948, some improvisations, and a reading of her manifesto on dance and life from *refus global*. Her subsequent choreography placed heavy emphasis on ritual and the principles of *automatisme*, and her symbolic, naive expressions of the subconscious helped bring Montreal dance out of the ghetto of American influence.

Iro Tembeck, the first of the Nouvelle Aire originals to break away to form an independent group (Axis, which she co-founded in 1977) also used myth-forms and ritual in her continuing search for what she called "primitive trance" in dance.

A cosmic ritualism is at the heart, too, of the work of Marie Chouinard, a young Montreal dancer who in the mid-1980s joined Lock as one of Quebec's best-known dancers abroad. In *L'Après-midi d'un faune*, wearing a skeletal animal headdress, she offered a modernist tribute to the dance heritage—an evocation, through her own esthetic filter, of what we know of Nijinsky's famous ballet. In *S.T.A.B. (Space, Time and Beyond)*, wearing a G-string, silver boots and a microphone helmet to which was attached a slender curving antenna that swirled and dived around her red-painted body like the headdress of a god in a Chinese opera, she grunted and croaked and made animal sounds. At first sight, her work is wreathed in a private mystery; but the disconnected episodes of rite and performance that she structures for herself make a dreamlike sense.

Ginette Laurin danced with most of the Montreal choreographers before establishing her own company, O Vertigo Danse, in 1984. The title was apt; she took the sky-flying risk of the Lock company one step further, persuading her dancers to defy gravity as they climbed and fell, swooped and dived, lunged and plunged, tossed themselves and each other through the air with what looked like a reckless abandon. A former athlete, she emphasized, like many of the New York post-modernists, natural or street movement, a sense of improvisation hovering on the air. But she also offered Montreal's romantic and sometimes humorous variant on New York's sometimes grim ordinariness. One of her early works, *Chevy Dream*, was an episode of flamboyant kinetic game-playing in and around an actual 1950s Chevy.

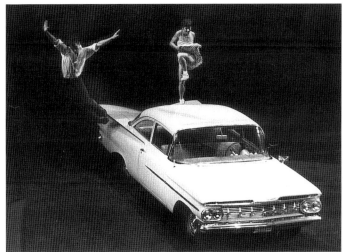

Ginette Laurin and Kenneth Gould, of O Vertigo Danse, in Laurin's Chevy Dream, *created for the modern dance gala at Expo 86 in Vancouver. (Guy Palmer photograph)*

Full House evoked in a wry manner the uncertainty and frustration of the 1950s through a choreographic language of tension and collapse.

Margie Gillis is an independent Montreal choreographer-dancer who has always existed outside the modernist mainstream. She trained in modern dance in Montreal and New York, eventually developing a romantic, expressive style that speaks directly and powerfully about social issues of an emotionally charged kind. Often compared in effect to Isadora Duncan and Loie Fuller, Gillis deals with her subjects in an effusive, heart-on-sleeve manner, using movement from a limited choreographic and technical range. Some regard her work as emotional blackmail; its strongest effect is often its musical accompaniment (popular singers like Tom Waits and Marianne Faithfull) and the use she makes of her exposed body and long, flowing hair; she is one of the few solo dancers anywhere who can fill large auditoria. In 1979 she was invited to give master classes for both the Shanghai and Beijing Ballet companies—the first modern dancer to perform and teach in China.

Jean-Pierre Perreault is regarded internationally as one of the most significant of the choreographers to emerge from the Montreal hothouse. Although he has always professed not to express any specific ideas in his work, there has been a clear trend—in his ritualistic and sombre treatment of the mass—toward social statement. In *Stella*, 24 identically dressed women executed a series of abstracted routines that demanded strict regimentation and hopeless obedience. Perreault called it "a subjective look at the collective unconscious," but there seemed to be clear messages about the balance between power and submissiveness—themes that have often surfaced in his work.

Not much of what happened in Montreal dance in the 1980s was entirely new, or even unique to Montreal, but it was an expression of the spirit of its time and place. Its hard-eyed views of society were tinged with poetry and innocence—an attitude that derived, perhaps, from Montreal's Gallic fascination with the lyrical and the beautiful, from its determined belief in the sanctity of individual expression, and from an inability, despite all the best efforts of the post-modernists, to discard entirely the relationship between dance and the poetic tradition.

In 1987 Paul-André Fortier joined forces with former Grands Ballets dancer and co-artistic director Daniel Jackson to launch Montréal Danse—a permanent showcase for original works by the principal elements of the Montreal modernist explosion and by international leaders of dance modernism—but in 1989 resumed direction of a company under his own name.

At the same time, the leaders of the modernist pack began to demonstrate a new fascination with technical excellence as well as instant theatrical impact. The impetus to outrageousness was undiminished, but a new discipline was apparent. Lock began to overlay the kinetic shock of his airborne crash-dance with a new choreographic, even balletic substance. Laurin began to probe new expressive depths. Fortier began to create work that synthesized the sensibilities of the time with a new and subtle exactness. The movement was finding the beginnings of a courageous new maturity.

HUNGRY YOUNG TIGERS

In the 1980s some of the most advanced and exciting creative work in the performing arts in Canada was happening in the field of modern dance.

It was happening not in the country's modern-dance "establishment" (the handful of companies that had managed to infiltrate the Canada Council's operating-grant citadel in the balmy days before the economic portcullis was dropped, and were now beginning to suffer a hardening of the creative arteries) but in the grubby studios, community halls and converted churches that housed the growing community of independent and experimental choreographers.

But what separated these two camps wasn't just a matter of money. There was a growing desire on the part of young dance-makers to control their own destinies. The company system, with its emphasis on administration, balanced budgets and corporate responsibility, held no attractions. They wanted to give their energies to their work. And it was a different kind of work. They were discovering they wanted to explore areas that might not fit conventional definitions of dance at all. The post-modernists had opened up new possibilities: by the early 1980s the confusion between dance, theatre and performance had become acute. Some of these eager young tigers found a sympathetic refuge at the experimental art galleries, established havens for innovation out of which the performance-art tradition had emerged. And what gradually began to evolve was a form of networking, with individuals banding together for specific events . . . partly to provide more powerful grant-getting leverage, partly to share production resources.

At the same time, the Canada Council, recognizing the new creative significance of the independent choreographer, began to develop new methods of support. Vancouver's Judith Marcuse received the first grant to an independent choreographer, $10,000, in 1980; the following year the council gave a similar grant to Margie Gillis and introduced a programme of support for *presenters* of independent choreographers (organizations like Tangente, in Montreal, and Toronto's Danceworks, which since 1977 had been providing a space where independents and experimental companies could mount creations).

In some cases, groups of independent choreographers banded together under a loose umbrella, in the style of Toronto's TIDE, for mutual support. One of the most notable of these collectives was Vancouver's EDAM (Experimental Dance and Music), created in 1982 by a group of contact improvisers, new-movement makers and musicians, and showcasing work by individuals of radically differing interests (ranging from the high-impact, risk-laden contact-dance first popularized in Montreal to Dada-influenced dance of the absurd). By 1987 EDAM's core group had been reduced to four, with Barbara Bourget and Jay Hirabayashi breaking away to form Kokoro Dance as a vehicle for their own raw and committed dance style. By 1989 the only EDAM original left was Peter Bingham. The Rebound collective, formed in 1984 and presenting collaborative creations, sheltered another half-dozen Vancouver independents.

But more often it was a matter of individuals striking out alone. As the experimentalist star rose in Montreal, the city became a haven for choreographic individualism, much of it inspired by the success of the Lock-Fortier-Laurin group.

There was plenty of individual action in English Canada as well. Crossing the disciplinary boundaries in Toronto were several veterans of 15 Dance Laboratorium and the country's alternative spaces—prominent among them Margaret Dragu, a former stripper; Elizabeth Chitty, a performance artist; and choreographers Susan Cash, Jennifer Mascall and Terrill Maguire. In Ottawa a

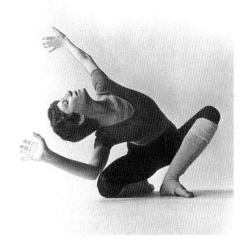

After training and performance experience in both ballet and modern dance in Canada, England, Europe and the United States, Judith Marcuse settled in Vancouver in 1976 as an independent modern-dance performer and choreographer. She established her own company in 1984. (David Cooper photograph)

tough and dynamic little dancer called Julie West caused an ongoing sensation internationally with her gritty, high-energy solos. Some, like Vancouver's Santa Aloi, a former dancer with Gus Solomons in New York, were able to buttress themselves with academic posts, though Vancouver came late to individual experiment. The city's first independent choreography series wasn't held until 1982, though close to 40 individuals calling themselves choreographers, most of them working in an experimental vein, took part in the city's 1984 dance week.

Language itself came under the modernist microscope, particularly at the hands of Le Groupe de la Place Royale in Ottawa and Vancouver's Jumpstart duo, Lee Eisler and Nelson Gray. Their work often dealt with the deconstruction of language, and they created theatre-dance works that explored the potential fusion, via new technology like video, of the new theatricality and the new romantic expressionism.

By the late 1980s, a number of new companies were beginning to coalesce around emerging talents–among them Michael Montanaro in Montreal(creating a vigorous and amiable variant on the Montreal post-punk school) and, in Toronto, Randy Glynn, a graduate of the Grossman company.

A fascinating variant on all this was Winnipeg. Like the Royal Winnipeg Ballet under Arnold Spohr, Winnipeg's Contemporary Dancers (directed since 1984 by former company member Tedd Robinson) frankly aims to entertain; it has a canny understanding of what its audience wants to buy, it entertains few discernible qualms about market pragmatism, and it openly borrows and celebrates other people's glitter. Robinson gave the city the *sense* of modernistic outrage without any of the danger, a synthesis of the essential elements of the post-modernist sensibility that was so prevalent in other parts of the country. He wore his influences (Edouard Lock, Robert Desrosiers, Ginette Laurin and Paul-André Fortier, from Canada; Lindsay Kemp and the German neo-expressionists from Europe) like fluorescent badges, impossible to miss. The company's audience (mostly the young and adventurous university crowd) grew to record levels.

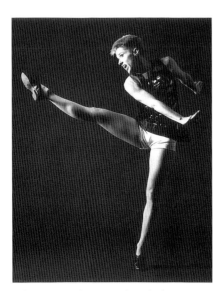

The New York Times *described Ottawa's Julie West as "small and wiry—a tough chick" during her five-year association with New York's Bill T. Jones Company. She went solo in 1984, touring North America and Europe with her intensely physical dance theatrics. (X photograph)*

Facing page: Sacra Conversazione, commissioned from David Earle by the Banff Festival of the Arts in 1984, entered the Toronto Dance Theatre repertoire in 1988. Using segments from Mozart's *Requiem* as musical support, it gives massive ritual expression to grief and anger in the face of violent death. (John Lauener photograph)

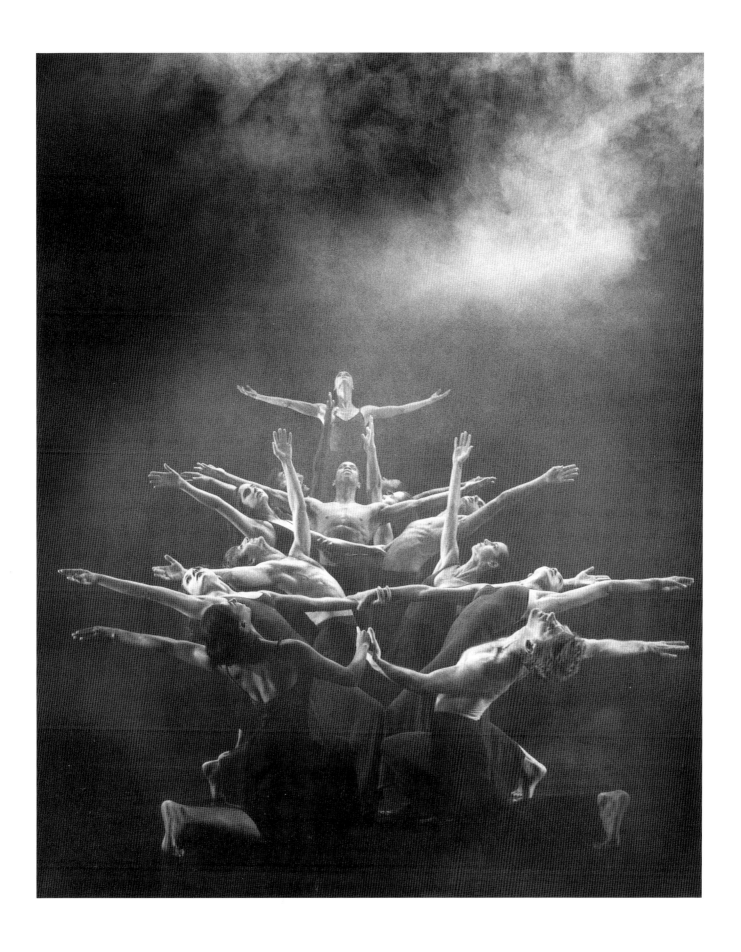

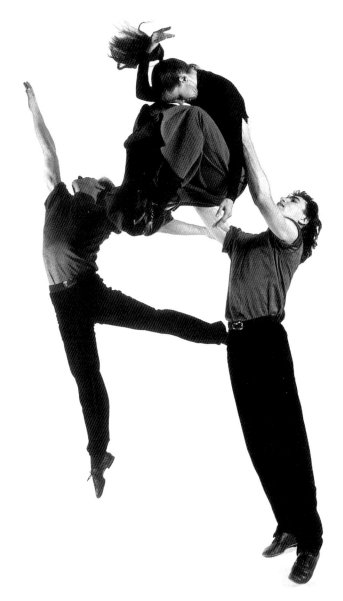

Christopher House, youngest of the four resident choreographers at Toronto Dance Theatre, made his entrancing pure-dance abstraction *Handel Variations* for the company in 1987. *Left to right:* House, Suzette Sherman and Michael Sean Marye. (Cylla Von Tiedemann photograph)

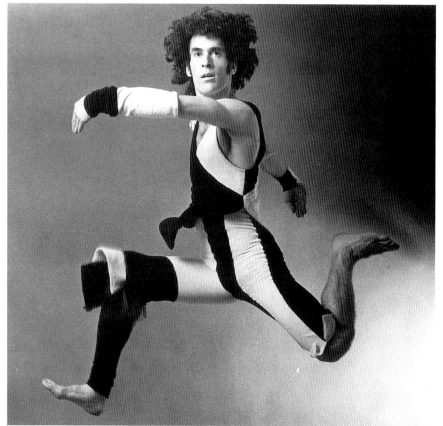

Curious Schools of Theatrical Dancing, Part One, made by Danny Grossman for himself in 1977, is an unsettling examination of the performer's need to perform and to be appreciated. Danced by a strange, harlequin figure entirely within a circuslike ring, it makes punishing virtuoso demands on the dancer's body. (Kenn Duncan photograph, courtesy Danny Grossman Dance Company)

Facing page: S.T.A.B. (Space, Time and Beyond) was one of a number of solo works that helped consolidate the international reputation of Montreal's Marie Chouinard. (Louise Oliqny photograph)

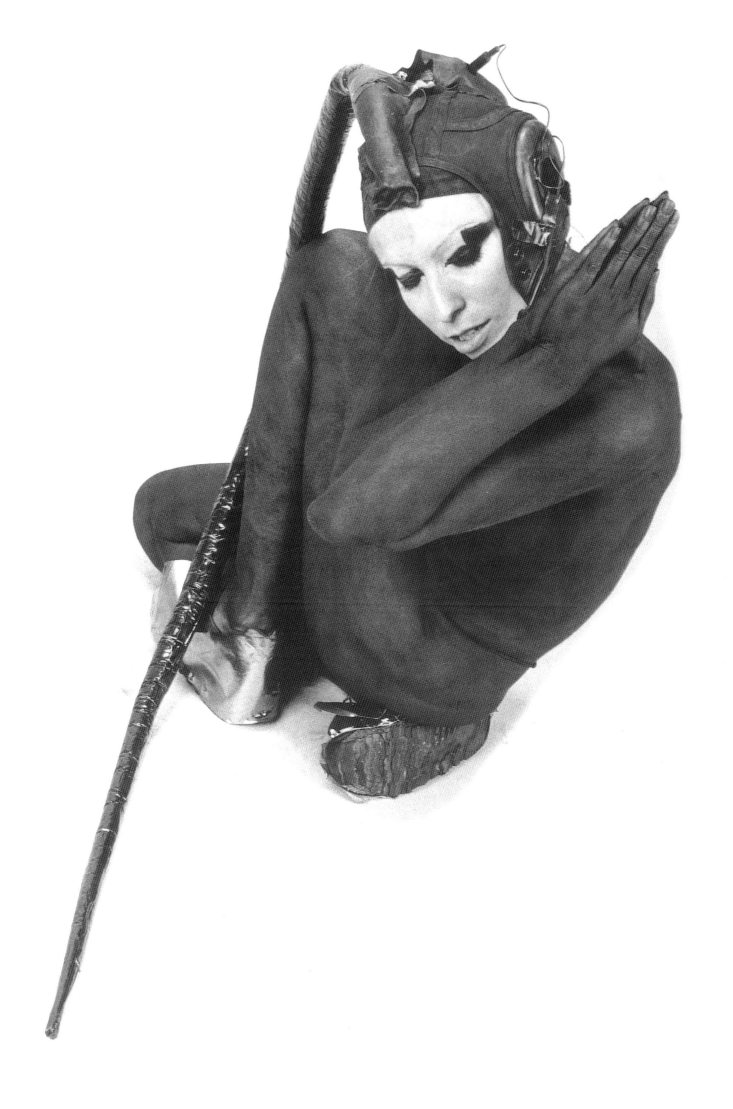

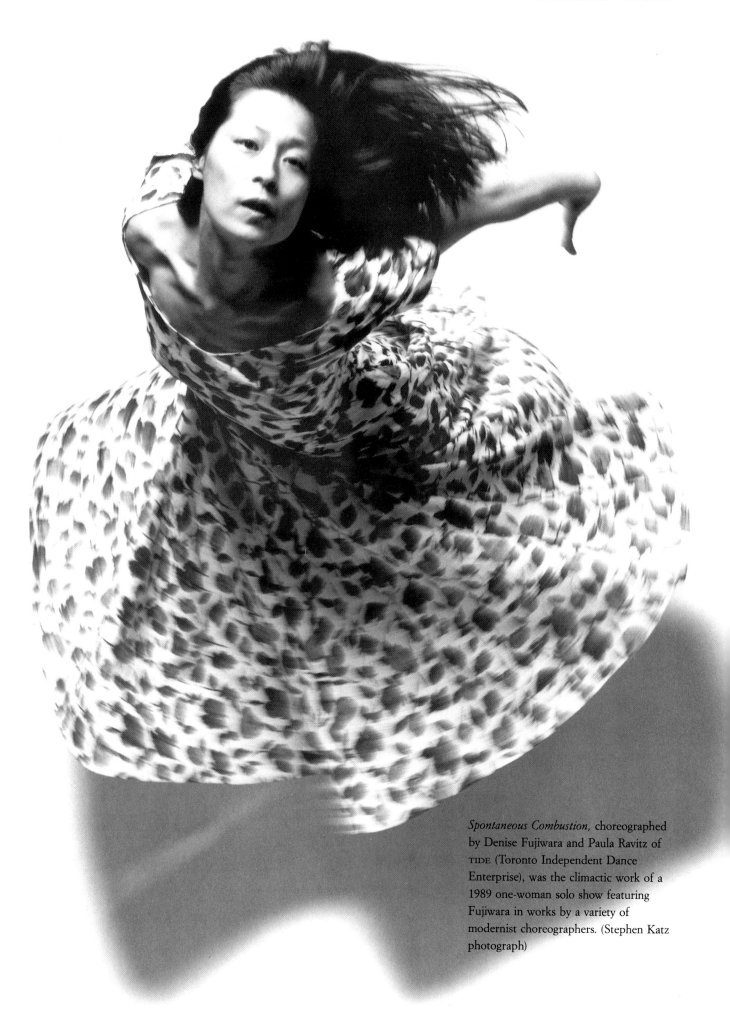

Spontaneous Combustion, choreographed
by Denise Fujiwara and Paula Ravitz of
TIDE (Toronto Independent Dance
Enterprise), was the climactic work of a
1989 one-woman solo show featuring
Fujiwara in works by a variety of
modernist choreographers. (Stephen Katz
photograph)

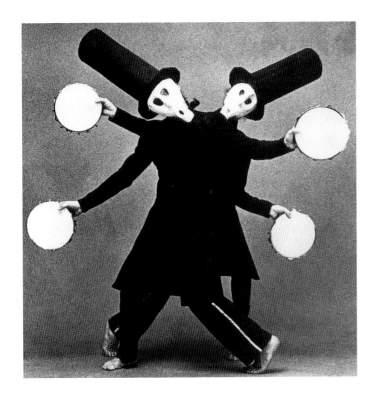

Robert Desrosiers established a reputation as one of the most fertile and audacious theatrical imaginations at work in Canadian dance. His choreography relied heavily on costumes and props for its sometimes stunning effect. This figure is from *Brass Fountain,* first shown at the 1980 debut of Derosiers Dance Theatre. (Frank Richards photograph)

Three Epitaphs by U.S. modernist Paul Taylor has been a popular work since its introduction in 1960. Set to American folk music, its mood mixes comedy and melancholy. This shows a 1982 performance by Toronto's Dancemakers. (Andrew Oxenham photograph)

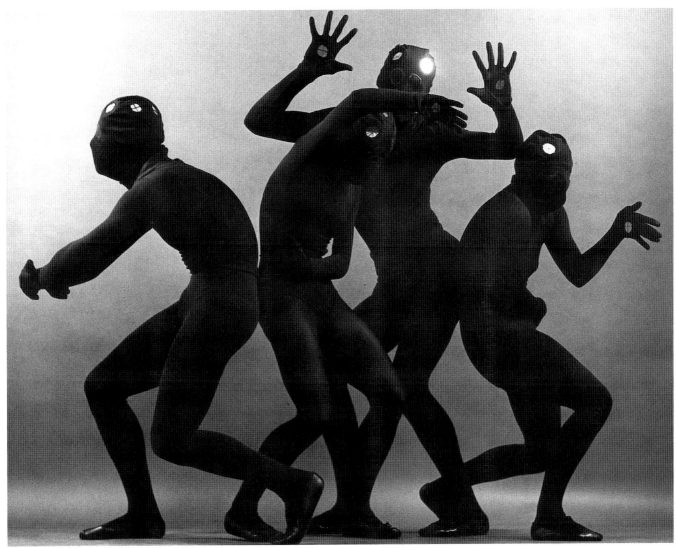

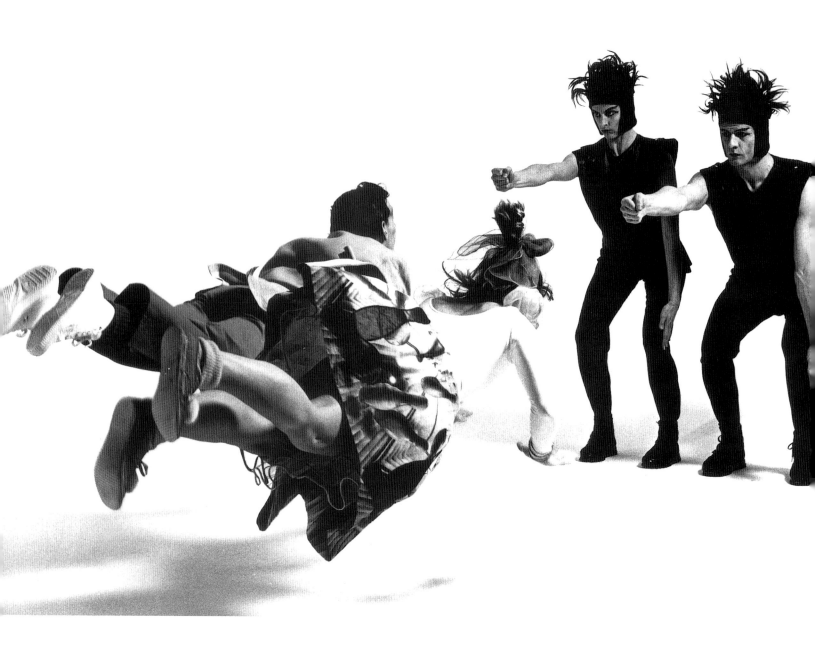

Randy Glynn's *Trumpet Concerto* was created for the Randy Glynn Dance Project in 1986. *Left to right:* Philip Drube, France Bruyère, Pamela Grundy and Glynn. (Cylla Von Tiedemann photograph)

Facing page: Dancers of Montreal's La La La Human Steps company, in a 1988 photographic treatment by the company's artistic director and choreographer, Edouard Lock. Straw-haired Louise Lecavalier (*left*) is the centrepiece of much of Lock's high-risk movement theatre. (Edouard Lock photograph)

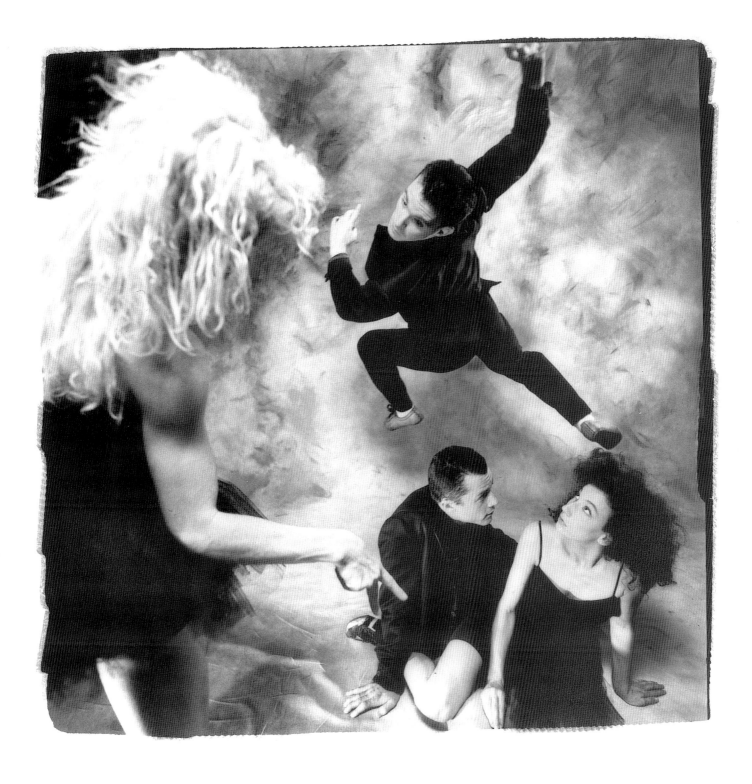

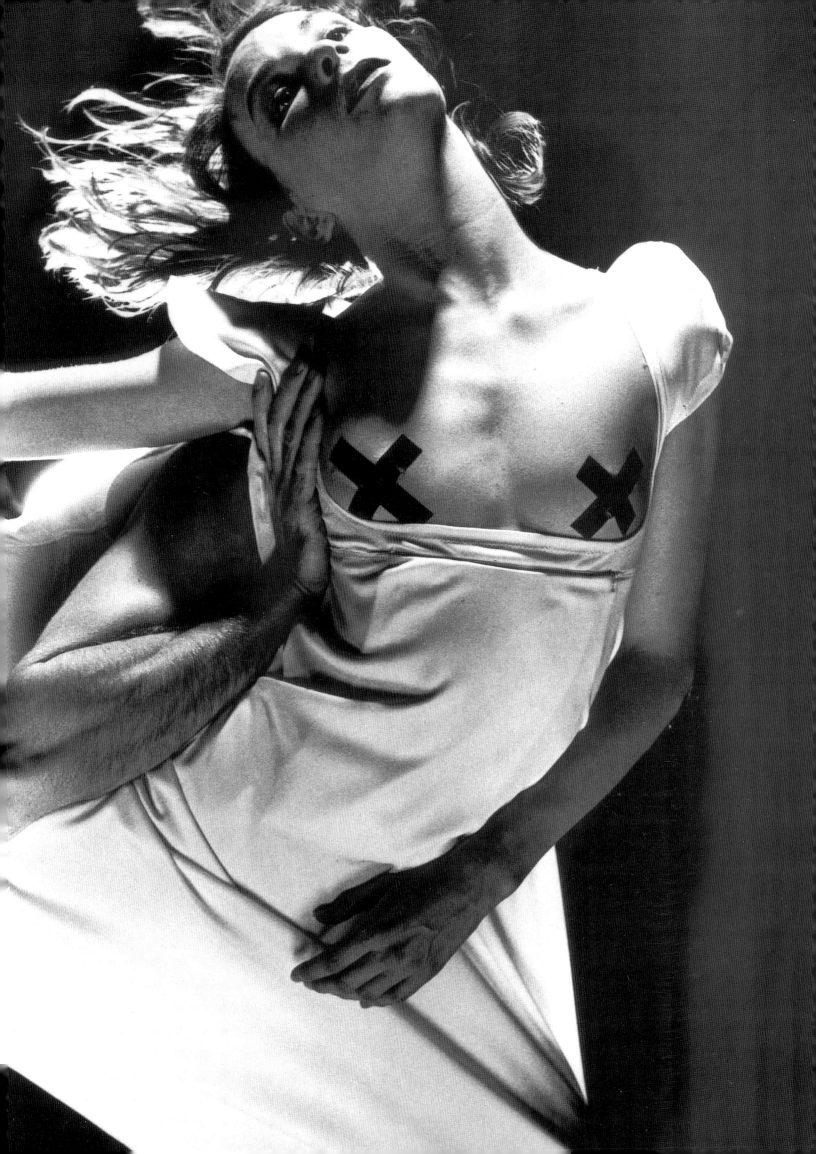

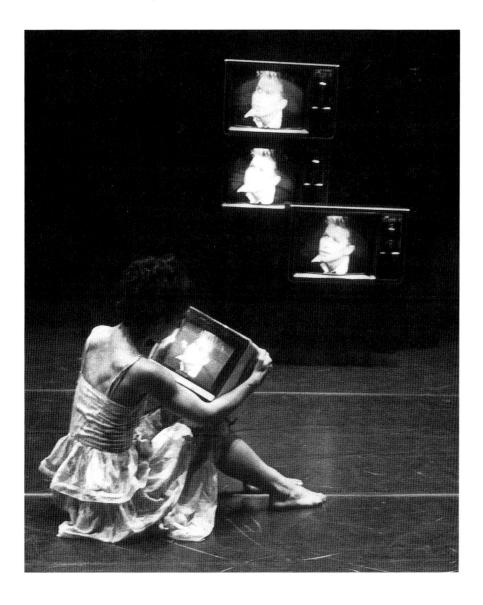

Facing page: Louise Bedard, with Daniel Soulières, in Paul-André Fortier's *Création*, a 1982 work for Fortier Danse Création that was part of a trilogy of dances that used rocks as images—of burdens, obligations, sterility. (Jack Udashkin photograph)

In 1988 Le Groupe de la Place Royale introduced its Dance Laboratory, where choreographers and dancers could explore ideas without performance deadlines. Peter Boneham's *Duet 2*, an attempt to integrate dance and video, was shown at a Laboratory open house. Dancers: Davida Monk, with Marc Daigle on the monitor. (Susan Close-Holden photograph)

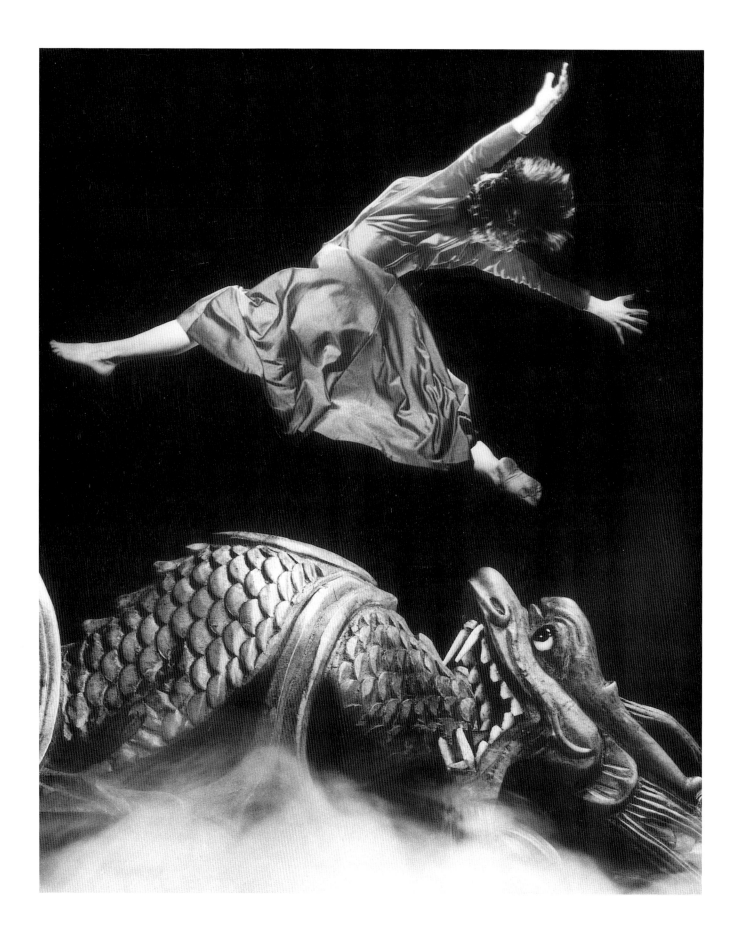

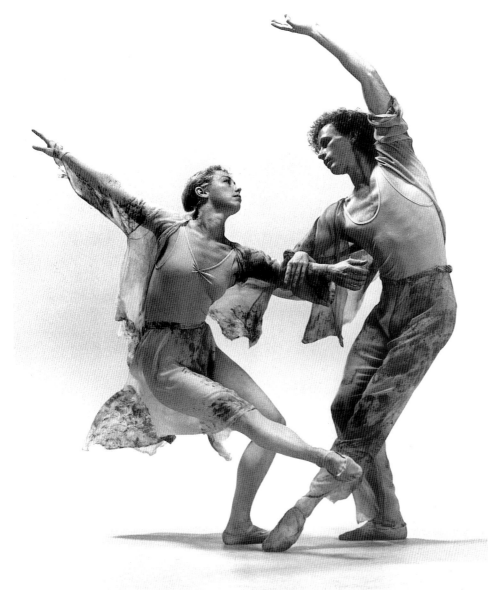

Facing page: Karen Jamieson in *Red Madonna,* a work she made in 1982, in the period between leaving Terminal City Dance and setting up her own company. Danced to unaccompanied spiritual-style carols, the piece is an intense, ecstatic response to the music's celebration of motherhood. (Chris Randle photograph)

Debbie Wilson and Aaron Shields of the Judith Marcuse Dance Company in *Seascape,* a work made by Marcuse for Les Grands Ballets Canadiens in 1983 and later taken into her own company in revised form. (David Cooper photograph)

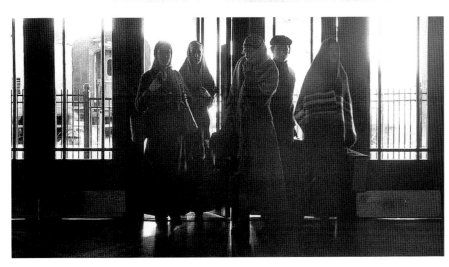

Publicity still for *Tales from the Terminal City,* a 1977 presentation by Vancouver's Terminal City Dance. Company members (*left to right*): Marion-Lea Dahl, Karen (Rimmer) Jamieson, Peggy Florin, Terry Hunter and Savannah Walling. (Chris Dahl photograph)

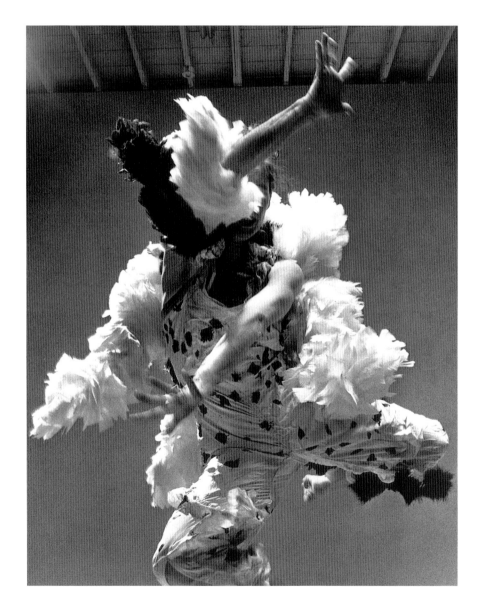

Independent choreographer Jennifer Mascall emerged from York University's dance program in 1974. Her work is characterized by an unwillingness to settle for established concepts of what dance might be. After seven years as a co-artistic director of Vancouver's EDAM (Experimental Dance and Music) company, she established the Jennifer Mascall Dancers in 1989. (David Cooper photograph)

Facing page: Dancers Fiona Drinnan and D'Anne Kuby are *Camping Out,* a 1987 work choreographed and conceived by Contemporary Dancers' Tedd Robinson, with choreographic contributions from Murray Darroch and Rachel Browne. (Otto Hammer photograph)

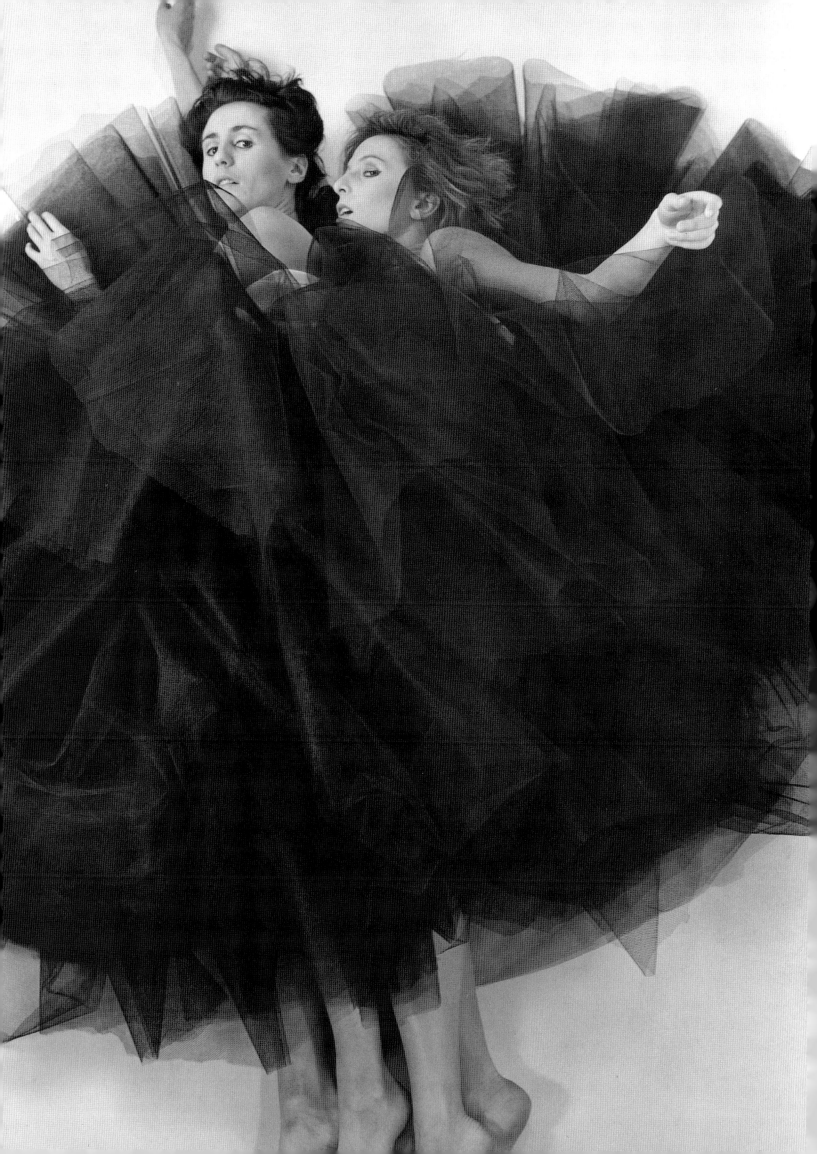

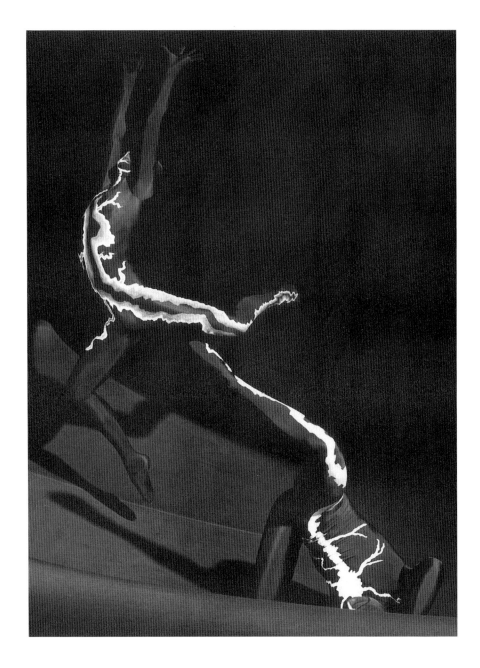

Anna Wyman's *Adastra,* a 1982 work for Vancouver's Anna Wyman Dance Theatre. Set to music by Jean Michel Jarre, with handpainted costumes by Frits Jacobsen, it created, said one critic, "an inter-galactic fantasy." (Rodney Polden Photographics)

Facing page: Peter Bingham made *Critical Mass* for Vancouver's EDAM (Experimental Dance and Music) company in 1989. Poet Gerry Gilbert (*top*) read from his works as the dancers performed. (Chris Randle photograph)

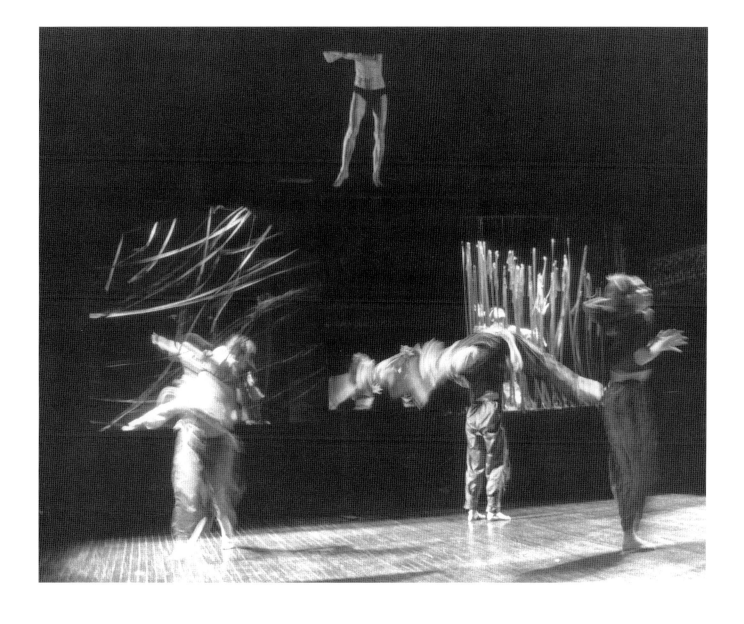

Conclusion: INTO THE FUTURE

By the end of the 1980s, there were new faces at the head of all three of the major ballet companies—and in each case, the old definitions became outdated as new company identities evolved.

Erik Bruhn's successors at the National Ballet, Valerie Wilder and Lynn Wallis, had both been intimately involved in Bruhn's hopes and plans, and—with the assistance of Glen Tetley as artistic advisor—they struggled valiantly in the years immediately following Bruhn's death to complete the transition he had initiated. But while performance standards stayed high, it was soon possible to discern in the repertoire the worrying beginnings of a retreat into conservatism from the outer reaches of experiment and excitement toward which Bruhn had been moving.

In 1988 the National Ballet board announced that artistic direction would be assumed by Reid Anderson, the Canadian who had returned home in 1987 after a distinguished career with the Stuttgart Ballet to direct Ballet B.C. in Vancouver. While promising to maintain and develop the National Ballet's classical base, Anderson made it clear that he also wanted to extend the company's modern-ballet repertoire. Through his Stuttgart connections he has access to all the Cranko repertoire, and his introduction of works by Cranko and a number of prominent German choreographers to the repertoire of Ballet B.C. was a major reason for the Vancouver company's rapid rise.

In Winnipeg, Arnold Spohr finally stepped down after 30 years as artistic director of the Royal Winnipeg Ballet in the summer of 1988. He was succeeded by Henny Jurriens, the former Dutch National Ballet principal who had been a guest in Winnipeg for several seasons. Jurriens claimed he would not make any radical changes in the company's artistic direction—"Why cut down a healthy tree?" he asked. But it seemed likely that his long-established connections with the Dutch school of ballet would continue to move the company toward European modernism and away from the crowd-pleasing pop-ballets that had always been a part of its eclectic appeal—though he cannily covered his bets by commisioning a ballet version of *Anne of Green Gables* for the 1989–90 season. This promised an interesting clash, since the presence of Anderson at the head of the National Ballet suggested the two companies might increasingly find themselves rivals for the best material from Europe. However, this promise was cruelly dashed when Jurriens and his wife were killed in an auto accident in 1989. He was succeeded as interim artistic director by principal dancer André Lewis, a member of the artistic staff since 1985.

In Montreal, meanwhile, the risky new directions in programming had been disastrous at the box office. Late in 1987 Jeanne Renaud left Les Grands Ballets Canadiens and returned to her university position at the request of the company board—ostensibly as a means of easing the company's deficit of over $650,000. In 1988 Colin McIntyre returned to a newly created post as director-general of the company, with Stearns as artistic director and Fernand Nault as artistic advisor. Stearns retired in 1989. She was succeeded by Laurence Rhodes, a former principal dancer with the Joffrey, Harkness and Feld ballets.

The company's ambitions in the area of new work were by no means entirely abandoned, but it was clear that if the company wanted to recapture its lost audience, it was going to have to provide more for the lovers of classical ballet. Accordingly, the 1988–89 season featured, along with three contemporary works, a new and lavish production of *Coppélia* and a programme in homage to Diaghilev, featuring *Les Sylphides*, *Les Noces* and the first Canadian production of *Petrouchka*, the 1911 ballet for Nijinsky by Michel Fokine, founder Ludmilla Chiriaeff's "Uncle Mischa."

——————

The face of modern dance was changing as well, but in a different way.

By the late 1980s, the modern dance boom was over. The audience that had "discovered" modern dance with such enthusiasm was gone, and a new, self-protective conservatism had become apparent.

Ironically, this was precisely the period when Canadian modern dance, forced for so long to clothe itself in borrowed styles and other people's traditions, had reached the point where it could display to the world the home-made products of its own originality. And no one was interested.

As cutbacks in government funding for the Canada Council steadily eroded dance's backbone of financial support, and the realities of the box office came to play an increasingly important role in an organization's survival, marketability became an increasingly important consideration in the creation of new work.

This sounds more like bookkeeping than art. What had arisen in the market-driven, lowest-common-denominator society of the late 1980s was a popular assumption that art (like television or newspapers or any other created medium of communication) should be instantly digestible and leave the consumer feeling comfortable, like some form of esthetic cocoa. It was an assumption that provided the crutch on which rested growing numbers of the walking wounded from the last great arts battle of the century, the battle between the defenders of excellence and the forces of populism.

Advocates of the populist approach argue that success at the box office deserves the encouragement of the public purse. The elitists argue that public popularity is no measure of artistic excellence, which is what the Canada Council is in place to foster. That battle is not yet over, despite what some pessimists suggest. But on its outcome hinges much of the artistic future of professional dance in Canada.

The debate has put those who are in charge of supporting art in a tricky spot. Art has always provided a barometer by which we might predict the changing weather of human history. A certain amount of avant-garde art is always concerned with changing the *status quo* of society—the advocacy of new regimes or systems, and the overthrow of the old. The seeds of social change can often be discerned in these artistic experiments, these accumulating rebellions. So as it as-

sumes more and more of the burden of support for the penniless modernist experimenters, the government finds itself increasingly in the position of supporting
revolution.

While the Canada Council's support has provided the economic climate in
which dance in Canada has been able to blossom, its methods and policies have
not always won unanimous support. Given its financial restrictions, the council is
specific about the forms of dance it will fund—ballet, modern and experimental.
Programmes exist for individual artists, schools, support organizations and independent choreographers and their presenters, but the council's chief support for
dance is through grants to companies, using as its principal criteria demonstrated
artistic quality, administrative competence and financial need.

Implicit in this granting structure is an assumption that companies receiving
support will accumulate quality and maturity in a linear fashion. Many do. But
there is a new subdivision of creative artists not interested in forming companies
or working within formal economic frameworks. Other individuals feel trapped by
the system; to obtain grant support, they have to show continuing activity and
steady growth. But if a choreographer wants to take a year off, or does not want a
company, or chooses to create only when it suits him or her, what then?

With its funding allocation from the federal government either frozen or
diminished through the late 1970s and much of the 1980s, the Canada Council has
dealt with these problems as best it can. It has sometimes assured an organization's survival for purely artistic reasons. But it has also from time to time removed
flagging companies from its support system on grounds of artistic incompetence.

The Canada Council has also begun to demonstrate a new flexibility toward the
independent field, recognizing that one of the great dilemmas for experimental
dance in the 1990s is going to be the challenge of reconciling the needs of the developing artist (including the right to fail) with the demands of the marketplace. It
has also begun to modify the expectations it imposes on a company like Le
Groupe, making fewer demands in terms of actual performance and supporting it,
instead, as a kind of dance laboratory, a place where dance's young tigers can go to
do their experimental research.

This commitment to Canadian creativity surely lies at the heart of the function
of the Canada Council. It must protect and preserve what is known and loved; but
it must also provide the climate for experiment and growth.

Much has happened in the years since the earliest pioneers of the arts in Canada
broke the first ground; but these stories of beginnings and struggles and triumphs
are clearly not the end of the matter. Against different kinds of adversity, the
country's poets, its playwrights, its painters, and the choreographers whose story
has been surveyed here, continue to map the spiritual face of this new land, Canada. The pioneering goes on.

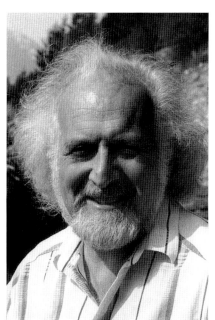

Susan Mertens

About the Author

Max Wyman was born in England, emigrated to Canada in 1967, and has since become a Canadian citizen. He has written and broadcast extensively in Canada and abroad on the arts, particularly dance. He is the author of *The Royal Winnipeg Ballet: The First Forty Years* (1978), and his writing appears in several anthologies as well as reference works such as *Grove's Encyclopedia of Music, The Canadian Encyclopedia* and the *International Encyclopedia of Dance.* He is arts columnist and dance critic for *The Province* newspaper in Vancouver. He lives with writer Susan Mertens and Mopsa, a Tibetan terrier, in Lions Bay, British Columbia.

Index

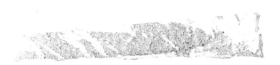